The Essential

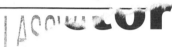
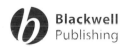

SECOND EDITION

Adrian Blundell

BMedSci, BM, BS, MRCP

Specialist Registrar
Health Care of the Elderly and General Medicine
Nottingham University Hospital NHS Trust, UK

Richard Harrison

BMedSci, BM, BS, MRCGP

General Practitioner
Windsor, UK

Benjamin Turney

MA, MB, BChir, MSc, MRCS(Eng), DipLATHE

Clinical Lecturer
The Churchill Hospital
Oxford, UK

Cartoons by

Rebecca Herbertson

BMedSci, BM, BS, MRCP, MSc

Medical Oncology
Weston Park Hospital
Sheffield, UK

**Blackwell
Publishing**

BMJ Books

D0280549

© 2004 BMJ Publishing Group
© 2007 Adrian Blundell, Benjamin Turney and Richard Harrison
Published by Blackwell Publishing
BMJ Books is an imprint of the BMJ Publishing Group Limited, used under licence

Blackwell Publishing, Inc., 350 Main Street, Malden, Massachusetts 02148-5020, USA
Blackwell Publishing Ltd, 9600 Garsington Road, Oxford OX4 2DQ, UK
Blackwell Publishing Asia Pty Ltd, 550 Swanston Street, Carlton, Victoria 3053, Australia

The right of the Author to be identified as the Author of this Work has been asserted in accordance with the Copyright, Designs and Patents Act 1988.

First edition 2004
Second edition 2007

Library of Congress Cataloging-in-Publication Data

Blundell, Adrian.
  The essential guide to becoming a doctor / Adrian Blundell, Richard Harrison, Benjamin Turney. — 2nd ed.
    p. ; cm.
  Includes index.
  ISBN 978-1-4051-5788-9 (pbk. : alk. paper)
  1. Medicine—Great Britain—Vocational guidance. I. Harrison, Richard. II. Turney, Benjamin. III. Title.
  [DNLM: 1. Medicine—Great Britain—Popular Works. 2. Career Choice—Great Britain—Popular Works. 3. Education, Medical—Great Britain—Popular Works. 4. Vocational Guidance—Great Britain—Popular Works. W 21 B658e 2007]

  R690.B64 2007
  610.69—dc22

                                          2006102502

ISBN: 978-1-4051-57889

A catalogue record for this title is available from the British Library

Set in 9.5/12 Minion, by Charon Tec Ltd (A Macmillan Company)
Printed and bound in Singapore by Markono Print Media Pte Ltd

Commissioning Editor: Mary Banks
Editorial Assistant: Victoria Pittman
Development Editor: Simone Dudziak
Production Controller: Rachel Edwards
Cartoons by Rebecca Herbertson

For further information on Blackwell Publishing, visit our website:
http://www.blackwellpublishing.com

Contents

Preface to the First Edition

So you want to be a doctor? Have you asked yourself why?

Doctors have a highly privileged role. Medics are involved in people's lives from facilitating their conception to dignifying their death. Medicine can be a rewarding career despite constant concerns regarding hours, pay and working conditions. Consequently, competition for places at medical school is high and on the increase.

Deciding to choose medicine is a decision that has lifelong and lifestyle implications. Do you know that you will have to spend 5 years at university and then up to 15 years before reaching the top of your profession? Do you know what being on call means? Even more importantly do you have any idea what life at university and a career as a doctor will be like?

Look no further because help is at hand. Here is the completely unbiased, honest and unadulterated guide to telling you everything you ever wanted to know about being a doctor – and a lot more. From the initial application right through to training in your chosen speciality – it's all here.

We have written this book to help you make a decision about a career in medicine. We hope that you find it helpful. Personally we had little or no idea what we were letting ourselves in for. Lucky for us it was the right decision and we love it. Sadly for some it isn't. Careful thought early on should prevent this; remember there are other rewarding careers.

Life at university is fantastic, no arguments. Life as a doctor has great moments, but be under no illusion, it is hard work, at times routine and it can be stressful. Read this book and embark on your career with your eyes and ears open. Work hard but more importantly remember to take time to play hard.

Please remember that courses and application procedures change, as can working patterns and practices. It is advisable to check the latest information before applying.

Good luck!

Adrian Blundell
Richard Harrison
Benjamin Turney

Preface to the Second Edition

The NHS and medical school education are going through the biggest reforms, possibly of their lives. Often a second edition just requires a little tweaking of information and updating. However, due to the major changes, this second edition is in many ways a complete rewrite. Even then, there is still much uncertainty and continuing change. The NHS is scrutinised in some form or other, practically on a daily basis in the news. In general the reports are negative and it is easy to become disheartened. Morale is also low with regard to the financial climate, and many healthcare professionals find themselves without job security. Although there have been few actual consultant and GP redundancies, some posts are not being filled following retirement. The expansion in the number of medical school places has increased the chance of gaining a place, but there appears to be a reduction in the number of training posts for doctors, which could lead to greater competition and unemployment amongst trainees.

Being a doctor remains rewarding and continually challenging. Our original reasons for writing this book continue to remain the same – too many school leavers go to medical school, only to regret their decision in later life. This is mainly due to lack of research into what a career as a doctor would really be like. From a personal point, our knowledge of our future career was limited and the reality is extremely different to our expectations. All three of us are pleased with our choice of career, although have gone through moments of uncertainty, which continue. The purpose of this book is neither to convince you, nor put you off a career in medicine, but instead to portray the reality of training and working as a doctor. Life at university, although hard work, can be great fun and this can continue in your future career. Work experience in different environments is essential, as is talking to students and healthcare professionals. If unsure then consider the options of a gap year, or even graduate entry at a later stage. Try to keep abreast of developments even during the early stages of your career and try not to be disillusioned by inaccurate television hospital dramas and the continuous doctor bashing in the press.

Good luck!

AB, RH, BT

Acknowledgements

We are extremely grateful to the following people for their contributions and comments:

Abigail Ash	Final Year Medical Student Nottingham University
Julian Boullin	Specialist Registrar in Cardiology Southampton University Hospitals NHS Trust
Christine Bowman	Consultant Physician, Genitourinary Medicine Sheffield Teaching Hospitals NHS Foundation Trust
Tim Brabants	Senior House Officer in Emergency Medicine (Locum)
Torquil Duncan-Brown	General Practitioner Nottingham
Marcus Hatch	Final Year Graduate Entry Medical Student Nottingham University
Bryony Elliott	Foundation Year 2 Doctor Sherwood Hospitals NHS Trust
John Findlay	Final Year Medical Student Nottingham University
Rebecca Herbertson	Medical Oncology Weston Park Hospital, Sheffield
James Hopkinson	General Practitioner Nottingham
John MacFarlane	Consultant Physician and Professor of Respiratory Medicine Nottingham University Hospitals NHS Trust

Sir Peter Morris   Former President of the Royal College of
                       Surgeons of England

David Powis   Assistant Dean and Director of Teaching and
                       Learning
                       University of Newcastle, Australia

Zudin Puthucheary   Specialist Registrar in Respiratory Medicine
                       Southwestern Deanery

Gemma Wilkinson   General Practitioner
                       Nottingham

Special thanks also to Gemma for writing Chapter 19, Rebecca for the brilliant cartoons and to our family, friends and colleagues for supporting us throughout this project.

Chapter 1 **A challenging career**

The decision to study medicine at university should not be made without a great deal of thought. At the age of 17 years it is difficult to know whether you want to go to university at all, let alone study for at least 5 years. It should be discussed with family and friends but must be an individual decision. Those around you are likely to have differing views; parents and teachers may feel that medicine is a respected profession and possibly encourage you to take this path but some doctors may try to dissuade you. Whilst listening to this general advice, you must try and ignore these opinions and pressures and try to make up your own mind. Without experiencing life as a doctor, it is difficult to know what it will really be like. We all know friends who have avoided medicine following their personal experience with one or both parents as doctors. In comparison many students, after experiencing their own family life, do decide to follow in their parents' footsteps. Although relatively common, do not be persuaded or coerced into studying medicine by your family – it is YOUR decision and YOUR career for the rest of your life.

University is only the tip of the medical career iceberg; the remaining 40 years of medicine can be very different. Whilst this career can be challenging, rewarding and exciting, it can also be hard work, stressful, tiring and, at times, mundane. Have you the right personality, not just for the university days but also the longer term? The majority of sixth form students have no idea what university and a career in medicine will be like, and embark on this journey blinkered by this lack of insight. However, knowledge can be gained by talking to current medical students, career advisors, GPs, hospital doctors, and by reading books on the topic of studying medicine and perusing medical journals. It is also essential to spend time in and around a hospital or GP surgery, known as work experience or voluntary work.

Students have differing motivations for choosing a medical career: family tradition has been discussed, others have experienced medicine as a patient, some have an interest in science, a minority have wanted to become a doctor since the dawn of time and many just feel that they want to help people. It is important to realise that there are other jobs and university courses that would

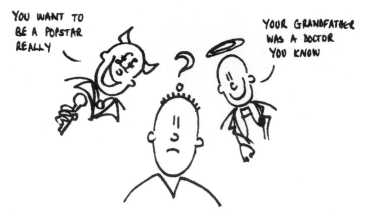

The decision to study medicine at university should not be made without a great deal of thought

fulfil many of the reasons that students often state for studying medicine; a life following one of these different paths could be just as rewarding. Remember that there are a number of wrong reasons for pursuing medicine as a career.

Once you are sure of your future career, you should check that you have the right attributes and qualities. Although academic excellence does not always equate to good clinical skills as a doctor, there are minimum requirements for entry into medical school. If you are not likely to get high grades at A level, it is unlikely that you will be offered a place to study medicine, as there is great competition for places. Apart from academic pursuits, it is important that applicants demonstrate other interests and abilities. Many potential candidates will have a history of sporting or musical interests and

---

Possible advantages to a career in medicine

- Five years at university
- Almost guaranteed a job following qualification
- Reasonable salary
- Diverse range of specialities
- Respected profession
- A job for life
- Opportunity to work in a team
- Sociable work environment
- Structured career
- Opportunity to work abroad

these attributes can be important. However, we do not recommend commencing a new hobby for the sake of it, immediately prior to applying!

Whilst deciding upon a medical career, it is important not to be disillusioned by the negative media publicity or the drama depicted in television programmes; these are two ends of an extensive spectrum and the majority of the work of a doctor can be routine. In terms of adverse publicity: doctors have not just started to make mistakes; doctors probably make fewer mistakes now than ever before; the difference is in the expectation and knowledge of the general public. Mistakes are now less tolerated and with the advent of the Internet, patients are more aware of their diseases and also treatment options.

Possible disadvantages to a career in medicine

- Five years at university
- Long hours
- Continued medical education
- Postgraduate exams
- Risk of mistakes
- Stressful times
- Dealing with death/suffering
- Patient expectations
- Media bashing
- Paperwork
- Lack of NHS funding
- Possible job insecurity
- Lack of flexibility in training
- Litigation (being sued)

Some colleagues may well know that it is their destiny to become a brain surgeon but the odds are that these people will change their minds over the forthcoming years. The idea of a speciality is different to the reality. For many the final decision to study medicine will be made shortly before sending off the UCAS (University and College Admission Service) form. This decision should be made only after careful thought and research about the career ahead. As previously mentioned, academic success is important but do not be disillusioned if your predicted A level grades are lower than necessary. Remember that these are a prediction following one set of exams. Once the decision to study medicine has been made, then follow through by completing the application process. It is still possible to be invited for interview and gain an offer of a place. Once this has been achieved, now is the time to study hard to gain the grades required (usually a combination of A and B grades). If a candidate is unsuccessful in obtaining an offer then it is still important to concentrate on gaining good A level grades. Once the results are published in August it may be possible to find a place at university through the clearing process. This is unusual in the case of medicine but certainly not impossible. A different degree course could be chosen and it may then be possible to change to medicine at a later date. Alternatively it is now possible to apply to a graduate entry course following a first degree. The final option would be to embark on a year off (gap year) and reapply to your chosen universities with your A level grades known.

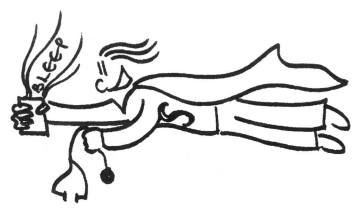

The job of a doctor can be challenging, rewarding, exciting...

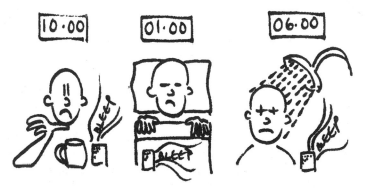

...but also hard work, stressful, boring and routine

The decision to study medicine is just the beginning. Now it is necessary to decide which university and, for some students, which country. It is likely you will have a great time whichever institution you end up studying at. Remember that not all universities are the same and at some the workload could be greater and the social life less. This is why research before applying could save heartache later. Once at medical school, the majority of those students who wish to become doctors do eventually make it through. Some decide that medicine is not the career for them and either leave or change to another degree. Likewise some students embark on other science degrees and find that medicine would be more suitable so make the change then. If you are unsure about your future career, then a possible option might be to study at a medical school offering intercalated degrees as part of the course. For example, at Nottingham, the preclinical work leads to the degree of Bachelor of Medical Science (BMedSci), followed by a research project in the third year. After this a student could leave the medical school and pursue an alternative career with a degree under their belt.

1.1 A changing profession

Medicine and the health service are currently undergoing radical change. It is unusual for a day to go by without some mention in the press about changes in doctor training and cuts having to be made due to financial problems. Morale is currently at an all time low due to hospital closures and job uncertainty for many healthcare professionals. It is essential as potential future doctors that even at this early stage you stay up to date with the proposed alterations to career structure, training and NHS reforms. Although it may seem irrelevant at your stage in life, the changes may well alter your decision to study medicine. One interesting aspect is that with the increased number of places at medical school and the reduction in the number of training posts, we will no doubt see unemployed doctors for the first time. The days of being guaranteed a job following graduation could be over and there will be greater competition for employment especially in more sought after locations. Modernising medical careers (MMC) is a government-led initiative which has been introduced to make training at all levels more formalised. Following medical school, newly qualified doctors now join a 2-year Foundation programme rather than the traditional 1-year Pre-registration House Officer (previously known as the Junior House Officer year). More information about the current and future training can be found in later chapters. Our recommendation would be to keep up to date with the changes by viewing the British Medical Association and Modernising Medical Careers websites (see Appendix).

There is no one good or bad reason for studying to become a doctor. It should be a decision that a student is completely happy with and should not be made lightly. For many, a career as a doctor is usually enjoyable and rewarding, but there are times when it can interfere with personal and family life and this can be seen with the higher rate of divorce, depression, alcohol problems and suicide amongst medical practitioners. With the changes in working practice and the reduction in hours, the impact on personal life should reduce. To help make your chosen career less stressful, it is important not to bottle up emotions but to talk through any problems with friends and colleagues and to have other interests outside medicine in order to relax.

PERSONAL VIEW   *Adrian Blundell*

I do not remember when I decided to become a doctor; my first career ambition was to become a pilot, but was not supported by my parents. They felt being a pilot would be a terrible decision, due to the long hours and the frequent trips abroad and not one that would be favourable for having a family. My parents are not from a medical background and so possibly didn't realise the long hours involved in being a doctor. Nevertheless the idea of being a fast jet pilot was then out of my head. At school, I was fairly good at science and reasonable at the arts. The headache initially was deciding my A levels. Science and study medicine, or arts and study law. (This limitation in my choice reflects my naiveté about the possible careers available!) Science it was and medicine followed.

My school was not particularly generous to me when predicting my A level grades (BBC). This was actually fair, as my results in the lower sixth form exams were quite poor. The most common offer in 1990 when I was applying to medical school was BBB, and for this reason I ended up obtaining only one offer from a London college. Other universities I applied to wrote back with offers for other degree courses but I had decided on medicine and turned these down. I actually contacted the medical schools to ask why they had not offered me a place – one response was that I had not done any voluntary work. This might have been true at the time of applying but I spent a large majority of my upper sixth helping at the local hospital.

Results day arrived; I had achieved BBB. A difficult decision ensued as I had obtained the necessary grades to take the place in London, but I was uncertain as to whether I wanted to spend the next 5 years in London. I really wanted to go to a university rather than a medical school, so I declined the London offer and took a gap year (see Chapter 4).

(Continued)

(Continued.)

I was unsure exactly what to do with this year. I had no guarantees of getting an offer and would not find out for several months. An advert appeared in the local paper for a school leaver with science A levels to work in the field of cancer research at a local pharmaceutical company. I successfully applied for this position and then began the process of reapplication to medical school. Many of my friends spent their year jet setting around the world. Although a little envious, I still had the problem of finding a place at medical school and this prevented me from leaving the country for long stretches. On this occasion I applied to Nottingham University, as I had studied the prospectus and liked the idea of a more modern course. I had never even visited the city before, but on the day of my interview I decided that this was the place I really wanted to spend my university days.

Fortunately an offer appeared through my door 2 weeks later. The rest, they say, is history.

During a gap year, the choices are: work, travel or stay around your home town living off your parents' generosity. The latter is to be avoided and universities will not look favourably at this. Work or travel is the main question. Most students undertake a bit of both. From personal experience this is probably the best advice, although working for the whole year did mean that I had some beer money when I left for university and also a car in which to carry it. The decision is yours! Good luck!

Chapter 2 **The application procedure**

All applications to university or college courses have to be directed through the UCAS . It is now compulsory to complete your application online as paper forms no longer exist. However, the phrase 'UCAS form' is still used in this chapter as analogous to the online application.

Initially, the task of completing the UCAS application form can be quite daunting; after all, this form will essentially determine whether you obtain an interview offer and subsequently a university place to study medicine. Do not lose heart: everything in this book is designed to allow you to make an informed decision about your future career, and this chapter guides you stepwise through the application procedure. We will give you hints and tips as to how to complete the form, tell you exactly how the UCAS application system works and guide you through the form step by step.

2.1 General advice

Medicine is one of the most popular subjects chosen by undergraduates, and is also one of the most competitive. To be accepted to study medicine, candidates need high grades at GCE (General Certificate of Education) A level (or equivalent qualifications), a strong interest in the medical profession and good 'people skills'. Medicine is a profession that combines an intellectual challenge with a strong sense of vocation and contact with a wide range of people.

2.2 Timing your application

Application dates

Application dates differ according to your chosen course and, in the case of medicine, are earlier. For the majority of subjects, your UCAS application must be submitted before mid-January of the year in which you wish to enter university. For medicine, however, you must apply 3 months before this, by mid-October. Candidates applying for medicine are not entirely alone in this form of 'discrimination': those wishing to apply for any course at Oxford or Cambridge, and those applying for dentistry or veterinary medicine, must also apply early.

Late applications

UCAS states that 'the universities and colleges guarantee to consider your application if we receive your form by the appropriate deadline', i.e. if you send your form in after the deadline date, they may consider it but there is no obligation for them to do this. Our advice would be to *never* apply after this deadline without extreme extenuating circumstances. The competition for places is high, so any reason to reject your application will be taken, and a late application is certainly high up on this list. Give yourself the best chance – apply as early as possible.

Deferred entry to university

The subject of deferred entry, also known as a year out or gap year, is considered in much more detail in Chapter 4. If you are considering taking deferred entry, you must first check that the university or college will actually accept a deferred entry application. When applying for deferred entry, you must obviously meet the same conditions of offer as those not taking a year out. If you accept a place for deferred entry, you cannot re-apply through UCAS in the subsequent year unless you withdraw your original application.

If you do want to defer entry to university for a year, it is not compulsory to apply to UCAS during your A level year, as you can apply during the gap year. This can be useful if you are unsure of what you really want to study, or if your exam results do not meet expectations (a route used by one of the authors, no less). However, if considering a delayed application, we recommend that you talk this over with your teachers and career advisors.

2.3 The UCAS form

Completing the form

There are those who seem to know they were born to enter the medical profession, but many doctors, most of them excellent and dedicated, were not sure which career to follow until the night before the UCAS application deadline! The best advice is, before you fill in the form, find out as much as you can about medicine and the different medical schools. You can do this by reading university prospectuses, speaking to your career advisor and visiting the university or college. Talk to your family and friends, particularly those who have been to the universities or colleges that you are considering. It would also be wise to attend one of the available conferences held for 16–18 year olds interested in a career as a doctor. These are held in various locations around the country several times a year. They involve presentations by medical students and doctors of all levels from junior to professor. Many of them hold practical sessions and small group tutorials. The main aim is to give advice on the application process and to give a feel for what a future career as a doctor may be like. Although attending one of these courses does not guarantee an offer of a place at medical school, it does show a commitment to finding out about your possible career choice.

You should be happy with your choice of course and university before you make your final decision. Remember, you will be spending the next 5 or 6 years there!

What happens to your application after it is submitted?
Confirmation of receipt
UCAS will acknowledge receipt of your application, after which copies will be sent to each of your chosen universities or colleges. The selection process is discussed in another chapter of this book, but once complete, each university or college will decide whether to make you an offer.

Offers
You will be asked to decide which offers, if any, you want to hold while you wait for your results. The maximum number of offers you can hold is two. If you meet the conditions of your offer(s), the university or college will confirm your place. It may also confirm your place if you have not met the conditions but your grades are acceptable and there are places still available. If not, you will be eligible for clearing, when you can apply for other courses, including courses at universities and colleges where you have already applied and still have vacancies. Clearing is discussed at the end of this chapter. Do not worry about the prospect of clearing – again it is much less daunting than it seems and has a very clear role within the UCAS system. One other point worth mentioning is that UCAS has no say in the selection of students; it is merely an independent intermediary.

Application methods
All applications need to be made using the UCAS secure online application system – APPLY. More detailed information can be found at www.ucas.ac.uk.

APPLY can be accessed from any computer with an Internet connection. Most students will make their application through a school or college and in these cases it is necessary to obtain the individual school's log in (also known as a buzz word). It is also possible for individuals to apply. Complete the relevant sections as discussed in this chapter and then it is possible to cut and paste your personal statement from other word processing packages. The application can be changed at any time and we would advise printing it out to check before sending. Once complete and you are satisfied with the content, the application needs to be sent on to UCAS through a staff member who will have added a reference. Individual applicants will need to register themselves for APPLY and also sort out their own references and include these before submitting the form. Applicants can pay online or the school can be invoiced.

When you do apply, remember to print out or save copies of the whole form for your own records and check thoroughly before submitting. Always review a copy before any university interviews.

Completing the UCAS form step by step

Sections 1 and 2: Personal details

The first couple of sections of the form is purely concerned with your personal details and can be completed in a matter of minutes. Most of this information is used to identify you uniquely and to help in the carefully maintained UCAS demographics.

1 **Title/Name/Address:** Name and title are straightforward, but be sure to state how old you will be at the start of the next academic year. Your postal address is the address where UCAS and your chosen universities will write to you, so make sure that you use an address where the post will either be seen by you or the mail forwarded without delay.

2 **Further details:** In this section you should say who will assess you for tuition fees, or how you will pay for your course. Funding and money is discussed in Chapter 13. For students who live in England or Wales, the LEA (Local Education Authority) will assess how much you need to pay and the amount of loan you should receive, so you should give the name of your LEA. The fee code that you are asked to give represents whom you expect to pay for your tuition fees. Most applicants from Great Britain and the EU will be in category 02. The part on Disability or Special Needs is mainly to ensure that your choice of university can meet your requirements.

Section 3: Applications in UCAS Directory order

Just in case you are worrying, you do not need to put your list of universities in any order of preference. Again we encounter differences when applying for medicine; normally you can choose up to six universities, but when applying for medicine you can only choose four medical courses. This is very important as, if you give more than four, your application will not be processed. It is also possible to apply for two degree courses other than medicine, to make up your selection to a total of six, but this is optional. There is ongoing debate about whether this shows a lack of commitment to medicine, but the universities all agree that a candidate will not be disadvantaged by doing this. If you want to apply for more than one course at the same university or college, you must put each course on a separate line.

You will probably know by this stage that, if you wish to apply to Oxford or Cambridge, you must also complete an additional application form provided by them. Differences when applying to Oxbridge are discussed in Chapter 6.

Another important point when applying for medicine is that, when you start your medical training, you will be immunised against hepatitis B. Some universities ask for proof (certificate) that you are not infected with hepatitis B. If you think there is a possibility that you may be infected, you should check directly with the university.

In order to complete Section 3 it is necessary to know the code names for both the universities and courses. These are summarised at the end of this chapter.

Section 7: Qualifications
• Do not send any exam certificates or other papers with your application.
• You must make sure that details of your qualifications are correct.
1 **Which qualifications should be included?** The simple answer to this is: *all* your qualifications. It is likely that you have completed GCSEs (General Certificates of Secondary Education) and AS levels, and these are the first to enter here, but any of the following should be included:
• AS Levels
• GCSEs
• Intermediate GNVQs (General National Vocational Qualifications)
• Key skills
• Royal School of Music (RSM) qualifications.
In this section you are trying to convince people that:
• You have the aptitude for medicine.
• You also have other, non-academic interests.
2 **What qualifications do I need to be considered for medical school?** The academic standards necessary for medical school are generally quite high, but there is a small degree of interuniversity variability. *Three* GCEs at Advanced (A) level (one being chemistry), or the equivalent level in the Scottish Qualifications Certificate, are the normal *minimum* entry qualifications for medicine. However, in practice you should have *three* A levels with good grades (A and B grades in most cases). These should normally be taken in one single sitting. All medical schools accept a combination of A levels and AS levels. Candidates with the Scottish Certificate intending to apply to universities outside Scotland should check the entry qualifications with each university.

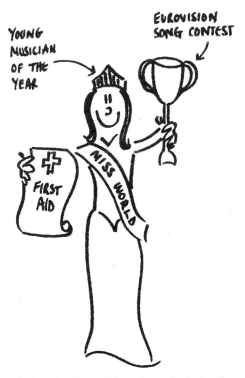

What qualifications do I need to be considered for medical school?

All medical schools usually insist that candidates have an A or AS level in chemistry and normally require a second subject to be in mathematics, physics or biology. The third A level can be in any subject, although most candidates take a science subject. Most universities will not discriminate if a candidate has chosen an art, language or humanity subject as their third A level as this offers a broader perspective. Occasionally, candidates with two art or humanity A levels might be accepted, provided they have the relevant science subjects at GCSE. It is not compulsory to be studying A level biology to gain an offer and there is no disadvantage to starting medical school without it. Such candidates will usually be offered extra lectures and within a couple of months students will be up to speed.

It is very important to check each institution to find out whether your subject combination is acceptable. Some medical schools will not accept general studies, art, music, design, media studies, home economics, and physical education as a third subject.

It is also important to have good grades (this means A or A*) at GCSE. Subjects should include mathematics, physics, chemistry, biology and English language. If one of the key science subjects (chemistry, physics, biology, mathematics) is not being taken at A level, candidates must have those subjects at GCSE level. Dual award sciences are acceptable at most medical schools as an alternative to the separate science subjects. Most medical schools will expect applicants to have a minimum of ABB grades at A level, but some (for example, Cambridge University) normally ask for three A grades. A few medical schools will accept C grade in some subjects, although this is unusual. In Scotland the equivalent qualifications are the Scottish Qualifications Certificate, or Highers, as issued by the Scottish Qualifications Agency. The Scottish medical schools accept a minimum of five Highers at AAABB but the English medical schools will require three Certificate of Sixth-Year Studies (CSYS) subjects.

It is important to check with each university for the required grades or consult University and College Entrance: official guide (published by UCAS). Please note that the requirements may change from year to year and having the required grades does not guarantee a place. You will need to demonstrate other skills and qualities.

As a general rule, the majority of medical schools will not accept BTEC (Business and Technology Education Council) or GNVQ in place of A levels, although about a quarter will accept a GNVQ, preferably in science (distinction required), plus an A level in chemistry. However, the situation may change in the near future. Most medical schools will accept the International Baccalaureate, European Baccalaureate and Irish Leaving Certificate. Some medical schools also accept Access Certificates, HNCs (Higher National Certificates), HNDs (Higher National Diplomas) and qualifications awarded by the Open University, but you will need to check with each school. The full International Baccalaureate at higher levels must include chemistry.

Section 7A: Qualifications completed
List all your qualifications in the order you studied them. Group together the exams you took at the same time and list the subjects involved. If you have more than one type of qualification (for example, GCSE and Intermediate GNVQ), leave a blank line between the different types.

Section 7B: Qualifications not yet completed
List all the qualifications that you are studying for now, and those where you are waiting for results. Group together the exams that you are taking at the same time and list the subjects involved. Qualifications that should definitely be included if you are taking them are: GCE Advanced Subsidiary, A level, Advanced Extension Awards and VCE (Vocational Certificate of Education)

Advanced Subsidiary, A level, and Double Award. For other types of qualifications, consult the UCAS handbook or website.

Section 9: Details of paid employment to date

It is likely that your employment to date is limited to a short time within the retail or leisure industries but, if you are a mature student, you can score points in this section by illustrating that you have been in the employ of a respectable company in a position of responsibility. Write down the names and addresses of your most recent employers, and briefly describe your work, any training you received (for example, a modern apprenticeship), dates, and whether the work was full time (FT) or part time (PT). You should include weekend and holiday jobs. If you find this section too small (for example, if you are a mature student and have had several jobs), contact the universities and colleges to which you have applied if you want to give more information.

Section 10: The personal statement

1 **Introduction:** Now we reach the part of the UCAS form that strikes fear into the hearts of the potential applicant, usually unnecessarily. This is your chance to inform the universities and colleges that you have chosen why you are applying and why they should want you as a student. Admissions officers will want to know why you are interested in your chosen subjects. A good personal statement is important — it could help to persuade an admissions officer to offer you a place.

2 **What to include?** This is one of the vital parts of the application. If your academic profile is appropriate, and your referee's statement indicates that you are not a serial killer, then it is all down to this!

One of the key elements of this statement is justifying why you have chosen medicine. You should try to elucidate your motivation for medicine, and any ideas and concepts that interest you about your chosen subject. Try to include any particular interests that you have in your current studies, especially those related to the field of medicine.

You should try to ensure those on the medical school selection committee that you know what to expect from the medical degree course, and the medical career that ensues. Include any job, work experience, placement, or voluntary work that you have done, and say how it has broadened your knowledge and experience of medicine. Whilst you should not undertake voluntary work purely to include on your personal statement, it is a very useful way of indicating that you have done some homework!

Remember that you may be asked questions at the interview that relate to your experience, so keep it truthful.

The skills that make a good doctor can seem rather nebulous at times, but certainly good time management and interpersonal skills never go amiss. These are the type of skills that you might have brought into play whilst obtaining a non-accredited key (core) skill that you have gained through activities such as Young Enterprise, Duke of Edinburgh's Award or the ASDAN Youth Award Scheme.

3 Knowledge about medical school AND medicine: Training for medicine normally takes 5 or 6 years. The main choice is between (a) a 3-year university medical degree course leading to a BSc or BA (offered by Oxford, Cambridge and St Andrews Universities) followed by a 3-year postgraduate clinical course, and (b) a 2-year preclinical course followed by the 3-year clinical course (leading to the Bachelor of Medicine (BM/MB) and Bachelor of Surgery (BS/BChir/ChB degrees) at the same medical school. Some medical schools include an intercalated degree within the 5-year course (for example, Nottingham).

The first option (a) takes a mainly theoretical approach and students have minimal contact with patients during the first 3 years. The second option (b) is more vocational and offers contact with patients in the first 2 years.

Not all medical schools follow the structure set out above, and courses will vary in their approach and emphasis. Medical education is undergoing major change at the moment with less emphasis on factually based lectures and more emphasis on student centred learning. In each medical school the curriculum will combine varying elements of traditional teaching, for example, lectures, seminars, direct experience, and student-led (problem-based) learning. It is important to read the prospectus thoroughly to find out what subjects are covered and how they are taught.

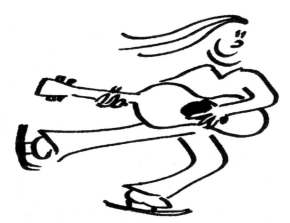

Candidates must demonstrate other interests and abilities

4 Work experience: Include all your work experience to date. Our recommendation would be that anyone applying for medicine should have at the very least been inside a hospital or a GP's surgery – and not just as a patient, although this may be difficult to arrange because of the importance of patient confidentiality. A holiday job as a hospital porter or work shadowing a doctor is always useful, as is voluntary work with children, people with disabilities, the elderly, or people with long term illness. Some people assume that laboratory work would be relevant experience, but most medical schools prefer students to have worked in a more people orientated environment.

When completing the UCAS form it is important to mention the benefits of work experience, for example, 'I spent a month in the summer of 1995 working as a porter in an Accident and Emergency unit in a hospital. This gave me the opportunity to experience the kinds of pressures that hospital staff are under, to observe treatments, sit in on consultations, and talk to doctors and nurses.' If you have non-medically related work experience, talk about what this has taught you. For example, if you work in a shop on Saturdays, do you have responsibility for money, or helping customers or managing people, and how do you think that these skills will be useful. In addition you should mention any courses that you have attended.

5 Schoolwork: Avoid mentioning that you enjoy working your fingers to the bone and that you read heavy scientific journals late into the night, every night. Firstly everyone applying has got good academic results, and secondly, unless you are really confident about what you have read, you may be asked a particularly tricky question about it in the interview – be warned!

6 Communication skills: Have you had a position of authority or used your communication skills in any activity?

7 Future career plans: It can be worth mentioning any future plans you might have. The majority of those people entering medical school do not have a clue about which branch of medicine they wish to go into, but if you have known for the last 18 years that you want to be a forensic pathologist (a surprisingly popular choice judging from recent applications), then put it on the form. It shows that you have future insight and have considered all the options. However, this could be a dangerous path to tread. How much do you know about the subject? If you know lots and have read widely and considered all the other careers, then it is reasonable to mention your career aspiration. If, however, you just spent a day with a psychiatrist, or just think it sounds interesting, then you may get into difficulties in the interview when they ask, 'What particular problems do you think face mentally ill patients in this country at the moment?' Remember it is not necessary to state at this stage which area of medicine you are interested in.

8 Year out: If you are planning to take a year out, include your reasons why you wish to do this. If you have already made specific plans, include these. The traditional way of spending a year out is to work and travel, but there are many profitable ways of spending a gap year. The subject of gap years is dealt with in Chapter 3.

9 Social, sport and leisure interests: Most candidates applying for medicine tend to have interests outside academia. This is important when the university is considering your application, because they are looking for students with well rounded abilities who have perhaps held positions of responsibility. Include all your hobbies and interests but the advice would be not to lie because it is highly likely that these subjects will be discussed at interview. For example, if you put 'I'm a keen fell walker in the Lake District', be ready to know a few of the names of the fells you have climbed and which of the lakes they are near! Musical and sporting abilities should be mentioned and grades obtained in music examinations listed.

10 Mature students: If you are a mature student, you should give details of any relevant work experience, paid or unpaid, and information about your current or previous employment. If you want to send more information, perhaps a CV, send it direct to your chosen universities or colleges after you have been sent the acknowledgement letter and application number. Do not send it to UCAS.

11 International students: If you are an international student, also try to answer these questions: Why do you want to study in the UK? Are you studying any subject that you will not have an exam for? What evidence do you have to show that you can complete a higher education course that is taught in English? Please say if some of your studies have been assessed in English.

12 Conclusion: End the statement with a few words as to why you feel you are appropriate to be selected.

The reference

1 Introduction: The next, and one of the most vital parts of your application, is mostly out of your control. Once you have completed pages 1–3 of the application form and signed it, you give the form to the person who will write a full reference about you.

2 Who should write the reference? Normally the person writing your reference is the head teacher or similar, but UCAS give guidelines as to whom this person should be: The referee should know you well enough to write about you and to recommend that you are suitable for higher education. Obviously, this person cannot be family, other relatives or friends.

The personal statement:
* Sell yourself but do not over exaggerate
* Brief introduction about why you want to do medicine
* Work experience
* Avoid trying to overimpress with academic commitment
* Avoid committing to a future career plan unless confident
* Extracurricular activities
* Concluding sentence.

If you are a mature student, this should be a responsible person who knows you, for example, an employer, training officer, careers officer, a teacher on a recent relevant further education course, or a senior colleague in employment or voluntary work. There are instructions available to the person writing the reference available from UCAS, but normally the person will have written many before.

3 What will be included in my reference? Essentially, the universities are looking for a responsible person to verify that what is written on the application form is *bona fide*. They are asked to include information about academic achievement and potential, including predicted results or performance, whether the candidate is suitable for the course or subject that they have applied for, and any factors that could influence, or could have influenced, performance. They will also comment on qualities such as motivation, powers of analysis, communication skills, independence of thought, career plans, any health or personal circumstances that affect the application and other interests or activities.

4 How is this usually done? Usually the person writing the application will not know you very well personally, but will have a dossier with all the information required to write your reference. All the pieces of information mentioned above will be available from your form teacher, other subject teachers and school attendance. This is then compiled and your reference is complete.

5 Can I influence the reference? The usual answer to this question is *no*, but in reality there are things that you can do to ensure that your reference is as good as it can be. The first is to ensure that the teachers think that you have the academic ability to pursue a medical career, and obtain the appropriate grades at A level. Their grade predictions will be based on performance in exams and in the classroom, so a good track record, particularly in mock exams is vital. The other key thing that you can do is to discuss your career intentions with the person who is writing your reference. They can give you an indication as to whether you are likely to have appropriate grade predictions. Whilst the person writing the reference will not increase your prediction, they might be prepared to consider a slightly higher grade if your commitment to a career as a doctor is strong. In short, talk to the people who matter.

2.4 Clearing

Freshers' week starts at UK universities at the end of September. Usually, A level results were released on 16 August and the UCAS university places clearing system started operating immediately. By 19 September the total number of accepted applicants (all ages) was 5.5% up on the previous year at 34 4478, including those deferring entry to 2002. The number of under 21s accepted (from all countries) grew by 3.8% to 275 206. Final figures are still to come. Oxford, Cambridge, Bristol, St Andrews, and the London School of Economics had no places to offer through clearing (for full information visit the UCAS website or tel: +44 (0) 1242 227788).

A rushed decision about which degree to go for, in the heat of clearing, can be a wrong decision. If you're up to scratch and can change course once at university, that's fine; but dropping out after starting a course is time wasting and expensive. Of course you don't have to go to university at all; for example, if you wish to start your own business, it is worth noting that many successful entrepreneurs did not attend university.

2.5 What are the medical schools looking for?

Having a good academic track record is essential, as medicine is a very demanding subject, but most medical schools want more than just academic skills. Typically, they are looking for the good all rounder who has wide interests. Anyone who comes across (either on paper or at interview) as an academic swot or as someone who is a bit of a loner may be rejected. Sporting achievements, an interest in the arts and literature, experience of paid or voluntary work, and general life experience are as important as academic achievements.

A survey undertaken by UCAS revealed that most medical schools are, above all, looking for the following:
- An excellent academic track record
- Evidence of a commitment to medicine
- A well balanced attitude
- Ability to think quickly
- A wide range of interests outside the curriculum
- Competence in communication and interpersonal skills (known as key skills).

In addition, it is important to demonstrate the following:
- A realistic view of the medical profession and what it entails (best demonstrated by work experience, shadowing a doctor in hospital or a GP unit, or through community work experience)
- Motivation, stamina and staying power
- Finally, good health.

Remember that medicine is all about communication – it's very much a people's profession. Academic high fliers don't necessarily make the best doctors unless they can offer other skills as well.

How are candidates selected for interview?

The most important selection criteria are: firstly, the predicted grades at A level (which should be a minimum of ABB) and secondly, subjects already passed at GCSE (grade As are expected). After that, the head teacher's reference and the candidate's own personal statement (Section 10) on the UCAS form are looked at. Anything that makes you stand out will enhance your chances. Not all medical schools interview and for these the selection will be done entirely on the information in your UCAS form.

A candidate needs to show evidence of motivation to study medicine. This could include practical experience of medicine such as spending time shadowing a GP or hospital doctor, or voluntary work. Other achievements to be mentioned should include: Duke of Edinburgh's Award, Operation Raleigh, sporting achievements, school prizes, musical ability, or fundraising for a charity. Disclose any interests or hobbies such as: reading, collecting items, making things, being a member of a society, but remember statements like 'I am an avid reader' are pointless without expanding further.

We have included below a couple of example personal statements. These are not necessarily the ideal statement but are used to stimulate further thought.

Universities, courses and codes

University	Course	Course length (years)	Institution code name	Institution code	Course code	Short form of course title
Aberdeen	Medicine	5	ABRDN	A20	A100	MBChB
Belfast	Medicine	5	QBELF	Q75	A100	MB
Birmingham	Medicine	5	BIRM	B32	A100	MBChB/Med
	Medicine (Graduate)	4	BIRM	B32	A101	MBChB/Grad
Brighton & Sussex	Medicine	5	BSMS	B74	A100	BMBS
Bristol	Medicine (Premedical)	6	BRISL	B78	A104	MB/ChB6
	Medicine	5	BRISL	B78	A100	MB/ChB5
	Medicine (Graduate)	4	BRISL	B78	A101	MB/ChB

(Continued)

Universities, courses and codes (*Continued*)

University	Course	Course length (years)	Institution code name	Institution code	Course code	Short form of course title
Cambridge	Medicine (Graduate)	4	CAM	C05	A101	MB/Chir4
	Medicine	5/6	CAM	C05	A100	MB/BChir
Cardiff	Medicine	5	CARDF	C15	A100	MBBCh/Med
	Medicine (Foundation)	6	CARDF	C15	A104	MBBCh/MedF
Dundee	Medicine	5	DUND	D65	A100	MB/ChB
	Medicine (Premedical)	6	DUND	D65	A104	MB/ChBP
East Anglia	Medicine	5	EANGL	E14	A100	MMBS/Med
Edinburgh	Medicine	5	EDINB	E56	A100	MBChB/Med5
	Medicine (Premedical)	6	EDINB	E56	A104	MBChB/Med6
Glasgow	Medicine	5	GLASG	G28	A100	MB/ChB
Hull/York	Medicine	5	HYMS	H75	A100	BMBS
Imperial College London	Medicine	6	IMP	I50	A100	MBBS/BSc
Keele	Medicine	5	KEELE	K12	A106	MBChB
Kings College London	Medicine	5	KCL	K60	A100	MBBS
	Medicine (Foundation)	6	KCL	K60	A103	MBBS
	Medicine (Graduate)	4	KCL	K60	A102	MBBS
Leeds	Medicine	5	LEEDS	L23	A100	MBChB
Leicester	Medicine	4	LEICR	L34	A101	MBChB4
	Medicine	5	LEICR	L34	A100	MBChB
Liverpool	Medicine	5	LVRPL	L41	A100	MBChB
	Medicine (Graduate)	4	LVRPL	L41	A101	MBChB/Grad
	Medicine (based at Lancaster)	5	LVRPL	L41	A105	MBChB
Manchester	Medicine	5	MANU	M20	A106	MBChB/Med
	Medicine (Premedical)	6	MANU	M20	A104	MBChB/MedE
Newcastle	Medicine (Accelerated)	4	NEWC	N21	A101	MBBS/Acc

(*Continued*)

Universities, courses and codes (*Continued.*)

University	Course	Course length (years)	Institution code name	Institution code	Course code	Short form of course title
	Medicine	5	NEWC	N21	A106	MBBS/Med2
Nottingham BMBS/Med	Medicine	5	NOTTM	N84	A100	
BMBS/Med	Medicine	4	NOTTM	N84	A101	
	(Graduate)					
Oxford	Medicine	6	OXF	O33	A100	BMBCh
	Medicine (Graduate)	4	OXF	O33	A101	BMBCh
Peninsula	Medicine	5	PMS	P37	A100	BMBS
Queen Mary	Medicine	5	QMUL	Q50	A100	MBBS
London	Medicine (Graduate)	4	QMUL	Q50	A101	MBBS/Grad
Sheffield	Medicine	5	SHEFD	S18	A100	MBChB/Med
	Medicine (Premedical)	6	SHEFD	S18	A104	MBChB/Med1
Southampton	Medicine	5	SOTON	S27	A100	BM/Med
	Medicine (Graduate)	4	SOTON	S27	A101	BM/Med
St Andrews	Medical Science	3	STA	S36	A100	BSc/MSc
St George's	Medicine	5	SGEO	S49	A100	MBBS
London	Medicine (Graduate)	4	SGEO	S49	A101	MBBS
University College London	Medicine	6	UCL	U80	A100	MBBS
University of Wales Swansea	Medicine	4	SWAN	S93	A101	
Warwick	Medicine (Graduate)	4	WARWK	W20	A101	MBChB/4

General notes

Some of the information contained in this chapter can be altered at short notice. This can include changes such as the addition or removal of courses and alterations in course codes. It is essential to check the UCAS website for the latest information as the authors cannot take responsibility if a candidate ends up applying for the wrong degree at an institution that doesn't even have a medical school. (We're not sure if you can become a surgeon with a knitting degree!!) The usual length of a medical course is 5 years. The courses in the above table that indicate graduate or accelerated are 4-year courses for candidates who already possess (or are currently studying for) a science degree. The courses marked with premedical or foundation indicate 6-year courses available for students without the requisite science A levels. The remaining course indicating a 6-year course reflects the fact that a BSc intercalated degree is a compulsory part of the training.

Specific notes

Cambridge: The graduate course is only available at Hughes Hall (campus code 7), Lucy Cavendish (campus code L) and Wolfson (campus code W).

Hull York: This is a joint course. A student will spend the first 2 years at either the University of Hull or the University of York. In Section 3(f) of the application form, indicate either for optimum consideration. If you have a strong preference you may indicate Hull or York.

Liverpool: The Lancaster based 5-year course is campus code L.

Newcastle: It is possible to study the preclinical part of this degree at the University of Durham (Queens Campus, Stockton). The correct campus codes are N for Newcastle and D for Durham.

Nottingham: The graduate course is run at the University of Derby.

Peninsula: Another joint course where the first 2 years are spent at either University of Exeter or University of Plymouth.

Queen Mary: The first 2 years are spent at the Mile End Campus with the clinical years spent at Whitechapel. It is necessary to indicate W as the campus code in Section 3(d).

St. Andrews: Following the first 3 years of basic medical science, students transfer to Manchester to join the clinical course (it is possible to apply elsewhere for clinical).

EXAMPLE PERSONAL STATEMENT 1

I have always enjoyed science and, for as long as I can remember, I have had a flair and passion for the subject. I intend to combine this in the future with my strong belief in the need for high class, equally accessible public services. Therefore I wish to study medicine.

I am strongly motivated towards the ideal of public practice and therefore in helping people to improve their quality of life. Empathy, dedication and team-work are the skills needed to be a doctor. I believe I possess these qualities along with the desire to become a skilled practitioner. Medicine also offers lots of problem solving, which is something I greatly enjoy.

I am particularly stimulated in studying Salter's chemistry course, particularly the application of its usage in everyday life. Biology interests me greatly as it explains the mechanics behind the human body and allows you to appreciate how complex we are. Mathematics and physics interest me as much of the course involves problem solving; physics also offers theories, which make me realise how much we really don't know about the world around us.

I attended a course for potential medics and, through talking to students and lecturers, I gained insight into university life and the way in which medicine is taught.

My commitment to supporting others is evident by the work I conducted with special needs children at a local school. The children were of ages 5 and 6 and had an array of disabilities. During my time there I could visibly see improvements in their communication skills and confidence. This was not only very enjoyable, but also a valuable experience as it made me even more certain that I wanted to enter a caring career. I have arranged work experience in my local hospital during the holidays.

Outside of my academic work I have represented the B team for football, playing as striker. I was part of the sixth form team that staged a charity event which raised £2000 for Cancer Research. I have participated in the school debating society and we recently debated the topic 'Should euthanasia be legalised?' I enjoy playing tennis, badminton and football, which keeps up my fitness and reduces stress. I am a season ticket holder for my local premiership football team.

I am a hard working, honest person who enjoys new challenges. I work in a local newsagent, which shows how I am trusted to handle money and can deal with people. I enjoy this job as it allows me to meet various people. I am approachable with a keen sense of humour.

It has always been my intention to go to university. I believe it is a valuable opportunity where I will meet new friends and develop both intellectually and

(Continued)

(Continued.)
as a person. I want to use my time at university to learn as much as possible and achieve my goal of becoming a doctor. I am ideally suited to a university environment, with my ability to mix with people from all walks of life, and because I am highly self motivated and focused on my future.

EXAMPLE PERSONAL STATEMENT 2

I want to study medicine at university because I want to help people. Using the knowledge and skills that I will learn, I can care for people and offer them support through the role of a doctor. I am intrigued by medical breakthroughs and how new techniques are applied to cure disease. I am also interested in forensic pathology and the criminology aspect of forensic medicine. With forensics, medicine becomes more of a public service related to the safety of the whole community and not just about the treatment of illnesses.

I have recently undertaken work experience at the pathology laboratory in my local hospital. I spent time in all the different departments with the laboratory and observed the procedures carried out in each. I especially enjoyed the time spent in the histology department. It was interesting to see how the samples taken during operations were dissected and made into slides for further examination.

I have been volunteering at a local special needs school for 3 months. I spend 2 hours a week in the class. I enjoy helping out with the children because I have an interest in special needs and it develops my understanding of what this means.

I am an active member of my local Autism Action Group. A member of my family is autistic. I help run a weekly club for children with autism, and I am now trying to set up a group for teenagers.

During my spare time I play the flute and the piano. I have been playing the flute for 4 years and I am grade 7 standard. I have been playing the piano for 2 years and I am grade 3 standard. I play flute in a regional concert band and we have been on international tours. Music has allowed me to meet new people and travel whilst learning a new skill.

Chapter 3 **Admission tests**

Recently, entrance exams have been introduced for most of the medical schools. These are evolving slowly and are likely to change in style over the coming years. To make it more complicated there are two different exams required: BMAT (BioMedical Admissions Test) and UKCAT (UK Clinical Aptitude Test). Different universities require one or the other exam. This means that you may need to take both exams. The exams are used in short-listing and in the decision making process by the universities when considering whether to make you an offer. If you are applying for a graduate entry course then things are even more complicated because there are 4 different exams. All of the exams require an entrance fee which varies between the exams, although you may be able to get a bursary if you have financial difficulties (Table 3.1).

3.1 BMAT (www.bmat.org.uk)

The BMAT was introduced in the UK in 2003 and has three components:

Section 1: This section tests generic skills, including problem solving, understanding arguments, data analysis and inference abilities. It is assessed by multiple choice and short answer questions over 1 hour.

Section 2: This section tests material normally encountered in non-specialist school science and mathematics courses (i.e. up to and including National Curriculum Key Stage 4, double science and higher mathematics). This is also assessed by multiple choice and short answer questions over 30 minutes.

Section 3: This section consists of a choice of three short-stimulus essay questions of which one must be answered in 30 minutes.

The exam is 2 hours in length (in total) and currently costs £21.50 for UK applicants. The exam will usually be taken in your school or college but can be taken in 'open centres' if you are not affiliated to an institution that organises the test. Full details, including application deadlines, exam dates and practice questions are available on the website.

Table 3.1 Entrance exam required by different universities

University	BMAT	UKCAT	None
Aberdeen		X	
Barts, London, Queen Mary		X	
Birmingham			X
Brighton and Sussex		X	
Bristol			X
Cambridge	X		
Cardiff		X	
Dundee		X	
East Anglia		X	
Edinburgh		X	
Glasgow		X	
Guy's, King's and St Thomas', London		X	
Hull York		X	
Imperial College, London	X		
Keele		X	
Leeds		X	
Leicester		X	
Liverpool			X
Manchester		X	
Newcastle		X	
Nottingham		X	
Oxford	X		
Peninsula		X	
Queens University, Belfast			X
Sheffield		X	
Southampton		X	
St Andrews		X	
St George's, London		X	
University College London	X		

3.2 UKCAT (www.ukcat.ac.uk)

The UKCAT was introduced in 2006 and is a computer based exam. All of the questions are of a multiple choice format and answered 'on screen'. The exam is divided into 4 sections:

Verbal reasoning: assesses ability to think logically about written information and to arrive at a reasoned conclusion.

Quantitative reasoning: assesses ability to solve numerical problems.

Abstract reasoning: assesses ability to infer relationships from information by convergent and divergent thinking.

Decision analysis: assesses ability to deal with various forms of information, to infer relationships, to make informed judgements, and to decide on an appropriate response, in situations of complexity and ambiguity.

Each component lasts 20 minutes and will be timed separately. There is an extra 10 minutes to read the exam instructions before the test starts. Therefore the whole exam is completed in a maximum of 90 minutes. From 2007 onwards the test will change to include a further component which will assess 'personality'; it will attempt to objectively measure qualities such as empathy, integrity, and 'mental robustness'.

The exam currently costs £60 for UK applicants. The exam can be taken in any of 150 independent centres in the UK and many centres overseas. Full details, including application deadlines, exam dates, practice questions and the location of the exam centres, are available on the website.

3.3 Graduate entry courses (4-year courses)

Some graduate entry courses use BMAT and UKCAT but others use 2 other exams: MSAT (Medical School Admissions Test) and GAMSAT (Graduate Medical School Admissions Test).

MSAT (www.acer.edu.au/tests/university/msat/structure.html)

The MSAT was designed by the Australian Council for Educational Research (ACER) in consultation with medical schools. MSAT does not test scientific knowledge and examines more general and personal skills and written communication abilities. The duration of the test is 3 hours in total.

MSAT is divided into three distinct components:

Critical reasoning: This section assesses reasoning, critical thinking and problem solving skills using 45 multiple choice questions in 65 minutes.

Interpersonal understanding: This section assesses understanding of people and behavioural motivation and reactions, with the focus on circumstances requiring empathy and teamwork using 55 multiple choice questions in 55 minutes.

Written communication: This section assesses ability to communicate coherently in a written form. It is assessed by 2 essays, each of 30 minutes duration.

MSAT is available at test centres in Birmingham, Bristol, Cambridge, London and Sheffield. Candidates resident overseas may elect to take the test in Melbourne (Australia), Singapore or Washington DC. The cost of the exam is currently £75. Registration opens at the beginning of September and closes at the end of October. The exam is held on one day at the end of November.

Table 3.2 Admissions test requirements for graduate entry courses

BMAT	UKCAT	MSAT	GAMSAT – UK	None
Cambridge	Leicester	King's College London	St. George's Hospital Medical School	Birmingham (considering adopting a test)
	Newcastle	Queen Mary, University of London	Nottingham	Southampton
	Oxford	Warwick	University of Wales, Swansea	Liverpool
			Peninsula Medical School (for non-graduates, non-school-leavers, 5-year course)	Bristol

GAMSAT (http://www.acer.edu.au/tests/university/gamsatuk/)

The GAMSAT was introduced in 1999 at St George's Medical School for their graduate entry course. It has now been adopted by other graduate entry medical courses (see Table 3.2). The test is in 3 sections and takes place over the course of a day.

Section 1: Reasoning in Humanities and Social Sciences
The section evaluates ability to think critically, comprehend and reason and is assessed with 75 questions over 1 hour 40 minutes.

Section 2: Written Communication
This component asks candidates to select 2 quotations from several on the same theme. Two 30 minute essays are used to assess your ability to constructively draw together concepts and express ideas fluently.

Section 3: Reasoning in Biological and Physical Sciences
The questions measure problem solving aptitudes with regard to scientific scenarios using 110 multiple choice questions over 2 hours and 50 minutes.
   (Biology 40%, Chemistry 40% and Physics 20%.)
   GAMSAT scores are valid for 2 years, but it is not possible to mix and match scores from different years. Tests are currently held in January but will move to September from 2007 onwards. You must register several months in advance (see website for details). The cost of the exam is £188.

Chapter 4 **The year out**

The aim of this chapter is to provide impartial information on what a year out (or gap year) is, how it can be organised and to help you decide whether you should consider taking one. Even if you have already decided to take one or not, this chapter still contains some interesting advice. There is much information available about taking a year out, but what needs to be remembered is that potential doctors are facing a 5-year degree course instead of the usual 3 years, and this has financial and age implications. However, there are enormous potential benefits from a gap year, which can enhance both your university and medical lives.

Traditionally a gap year is taken between school and university. In actual fact a gap year can be taken at any time and also be a break from whatever you are currently doing. It can be spent in your home country or abroad; working or volunteering; or merely travelling and seeing the sights. Those embarking on a year out have become known as gappers.

4.1 The initial decision

Will a gap year affect my chances of getting into medical school?

This is often one of the first questions people ask. Our answer is no. Indeed university admissions officers seem to be getting more enthusiastic about the idea of a gap year. If the year is used well, many tutors believe that students start university with a better attitude, not only having matured and experienced more of life, but often more focused and clear that they have chosen the right course. The important point is not to waste it. At interview it will be essential to show that you have thought through the pros and cons and made useful plans. A gap year spent living off your parents and doing nothing would not be looked at favourably.

Motivation

Students will have differing motivations for taking time out before university. The first thing to realise is that some will have considered it when first thinking about medicine, whilst others may be almost forced to defer, if exam results are lower than expected. After the stress of A levels, some applicants decide a break would be useful to recharge the batteries before embarking on 5 years of further study. Others organise challenging exploits in various parts of the globe either on personal adventures or helping others by undertaking voluntary work. As mentioned above, most plans that you carry out in the gap year will lead to increasing maturity. Whether your specific ideas will help with your chosen profession will depend on the individual. In general, students want to broaden their minds, see new places, learn new skills, find themselves or simply search for fun and adventure.

Whatever your motivations for considering a year out, feelings of both trepidation and dread are common. For many this will be the first time away from home and the idea of independence and fending for yourself is often more appealing than the reality. It may not just be you who has concerns; often parents can be worried, so be considerate (especially as they will be helping financially over the next few years!). On the plus side this is often a person's first opportunity to take control of a significant period of time, without the stress of examinations looming or other responsibilities pressing.

For those not taking a year off, there will of course be a 4 or 5-month gap between finishing exams and starting university and, although probably not sufficient for a full round-the-world trip, it is certainly a time not to be wasted. Unfortunately, because of financial pressures, many students need to work for at least part of this time.

What skills can I learn from a year out?

This obviously depends on what you do with your year out and can be divided into general and specific skills.

General skills	Specific skills
Self-reliance	Language skills
Maturity	Music skills
Teamwork	Industrial skills
Managing money	Work experience
Communication skills	Appreciate culture
Integrity	
Resilience	
Adaptability	

A cautionary tale

Whilst most people have a fantastic time in their year out, there may be some for whom things do not work out quite as planned. Firstly if you make the wrong decision, you may end up bored; extensive world travel does not come cheap and it is early days to be building up an overdraft. If your choice is to remain at home and work for the majority of the year, money may well be less of a problem but staying a further year with your parents may drive you to the verge of insanity – a further 15 months having to live by their rules!

Some people find work only to despise it, while others may find a beautiful beach in an exotic location, only to miss parents, home or their partner. On a more serious note, world travel, especially if you are on your own or in remote locations, can be potentially dangerous. It is essential that you check with the Foreign Office before planning any exotic travels, especially with the added recent risk of terrorist attacks. Forward planning is essential and travel with friends would be highly recommended. It would be well worth reading a decent guidebook before embarking on such a journey. These tend to be written by well travelled journalists and are full of tips for avoiding trouble and staying healthy. Good travel insurance is a must and make sure that you are fully covered if you are considering certain dangerous pursuits (bungee jumping off bridges, etc.). If you go off on a trip on your own, make sure that people know where you have gone and leave contact numbers wherever possible. To make you aware rather than put you off, some travellers do run into trouble. It is normally through lack of sense. Take the precautions recommended and keep your wits about you, remembering that drugs and alcohol can impair your judgement. The most common problems tend to concern health and often these cannot be prevented – the dreaded Delhi belly! It is worth visiting your doctor before leaving the country and check to see which immunisations will be required. Infections that are not common in this country have an increased incidence in other parts of the world, so don't forget the condoms.

4.2 The options

Whether you have firm plans or just a seedling of an idea, you need to decide if they are realistic. Run through what you want to do, where you want to go and whether your funds match up. Following on from this, decide on how long you want for each activity, but remember to think about your plans for when you return to this country if you are planning to travel. Bear in mind the feelings of parents and loved ones, and discuss ideas with them. Of course they do not necessarily need to give their permission as you are now 18, but it is better not to upset them too much at this stage.

The main choices for your year off are:
• Paid work or voluntary work, at home or abroad
• Travel and adventure
• A mixture of both.

Gap year ideas	
Adventure	Media
Archaeology	Research
Au pair	Sailing trip
Child care	Chalet person
Conservation projects	Summer camps
Diving trip	Teaching English abroad
Healthcare work	Tourism
Journalism	Working with the disabled
Learn new language	Charity work
Marine conservation	Round-the-world trip

Then decide whether you will go with an organised group or completely independently. If travelling with companions, work out an itinerary before leaving to save arguments later. If you are unsure how you will manage away from home, plan an earlier trip immediately after A levels to experiment.

4.3 Practical information about a year out

General
A year out can actually last for longer than a year, usually up to 15 months. For many, it is a time that will not be repeated. You could, for the first time, earn a living, travel the world or make a difference to other people's lives. Research into your year off choice is very important. If you are going to work for the year, then start looking in advance and scout the local papers for appropriate jobs. If travelling, remember that organising can take longer than you might think. If you are applying for jobs, you may have to produce a curriculum vitae, which is similar to your personal statement on the UCAS form and summarises your main achievements to date. Another new concept will be that of the tax man – you may be liable for income tax to be deducted from your wage during your gap year. This could also affect payments in future years, so be sure to keep all your wage slips and other important tax documents in a safe place.

For travelling it will be necessary to sort out plane tickets, visas, immunisations, finance, medicals and travel insurance. As mentioned above it would be worthwhile checking various web sites and guide books for advice. Visa applications can take up to a month to come through so be prepared. The other difficulty is that you may well need several visas if you are visiting different countries in a single trip. A useful tip is to photocopy all relevant travel documents – take copies with you and also leave copies in England with relatives. Remember to take the telephone numbers for cancelling credit cards in case of loss or theft.

Funding

This can be one of the main reasons why people are hesitant about a year out. Without doubt it can be expensive but there are ways and means to help. It is certainly worth considering the start of university when budgeting for your year off. It will also be wise to have some money to take to university with you. Travelling the world in first class will be expensive, but the majority of gappers will spend some of the year working and then the rest spending. A useful option is to undertake voluntary work. Many organisations will pay for the travel and living expenses including accommodation. This is a good way of seeing another part of the world without the expense. Don't forget that you will probably be worked fairly hard! Planning is essential at this stage: for example, if you do plan to go travelling, write down all the costs involved and then work out for how long you would have to work to save up this amount. Even if the job is working in a fast food restaurant, you can save a considerable amount of money.

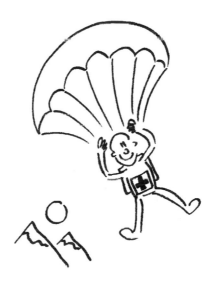

The gap year

Other sources of money include fundraising and sponsorship by companies or charities.

4.4 How to apply for a gap year

There are three main ways of applying for a gap year, each having a different strategy attached to them:
• Deferred entry (applying before A levels)
• Rescheduled entry after A level results
• Late application, also after A levels.
We would recommend applying for deferred entry. First of all, contact the university admissions department and find out if they accept applications with deferred entry. Whilst the vast majority of universities do approve of a year out, there are those that do not.

Deferred entry

Simply tick the box (having made the telephone call first) and wait and see. We would also recommend mentioning any specific plans in your personal statement. Also, talk to your teachers to see if they think it is a good idea. You need to convince the university that a year off will make you a better applicant, so give an outline of what you plan to do and why. It might be nearly 2 years before you reach higher education.

Rescheduled entry

If, after A level results, you have been successful in gaining a place at the medical school of your choice, you can negotiate directly with that university about deferring your entry for another year. Make sure that you check with the course admissions tutor in your first term of sixth form to see if this procedure is OK, before you make a decision not to apply at the normal time. When you have got your A levels, go back to the university and say you would like to take a gap year. If they say yes, you will receive a changed entry date confirmation letter, and you must send the attached form to UCAS within 7 days to accept the place. If they say no, you have the option to take your place or you have to start the application all over again.

It should be noted that this could be considered a risky strategy. Giving up a place on a popular course can be frowned upon, as the university may not be happy about being messed around. Others say that, if a course has over recruited, your deferral will be welcome. Tread carefully.

Post A level application

Scenario 3 is that you get no offers for the course you want but end up with the grades you need, or that you do not apply in the first place. You may not want to go through clearing for whatever reason, or find no suitable place in clearing. If you have your required grades, then when you reapply (if the university accepts you for your chosen course) you will be made an unconditional offer.

The only other option is that you need to resite your A levels, although this is likely to put you in a position of having to study for the majority of your year off.

4.5 Summary

Whether or not to take a year off is a personal decision, although the matter should be discussed with loved ones, teachers and universities. The traditional reasons for not taking time off revolve around the decision about starting university later and, as medicine is a 5-year degree course, perhaps you should just get on with it. Surely working for 45 years is not much different to working for 44 years in the scheme of things. It would seem that the benefits far outweigh the disadvantages. Of course it is an individual choice and not everyone will enjoy their time. Research and planning is the key as for most things regarding your future. Discuss the matter with students who have done both and get a feel for their various experiences. One thing that is certain is that it will change you – usually for the better. Added maturity, better personal and communication skills, and possibly new practical skills all add up to leading your way to a more successful university life and future career.

Chapters 13 and 22 also have information regarding travel planning and advice.

PERSONAL VIEW   *Rick Harrison*

Having been at school for 14 years, the prospect of 12 months of my own time, in which I could do whatever I wished, was quite daunting. At the time, there was relatively little information available on my options, but I had a vague idea that I would like to work and travel.

The number of work options was bewildering, with decisions as to which country to work in, what type of industry and for how much of the year. In the end, despite having a place at medical school, I applied for a job through a company called 'A Year in Industry', which mainly placed potential engineers with companies for a year prior to university. I had a job interview with ICI, working in a chemical analysis laboratory, and was very surprised to be accepted. I worked alongside existing chemical engineers and laboratory staff on a large ICI chemical production plant, and my job was to check the quality

(Continued)

(*Continued.*)
and purity of the chemicals at different stages of production. This involved taking samples from around the plant and analysing them for pH abnormalities, impurities and other criteria. I have to confess that day 1 was very worrying, when I was presented with a laboratory, told I would have 2 weeks' training and then be left to my own devices!

Working for a large company had great benefits, such as access to training facilities; I studied for a computer science course, for example. I also had great fun working with the other analysts in the lab, really experiencing a proper job for the first time. The money was good and allowed me to buy a car and have a good social life. The main downside was that most of my friends who had gone to university were telling me all their stories, which made me quite jealous at the time.

For the last 4 months, I set off travelling with a friend who had also taken a gap year. The trip took a lot of planning and also a lot of the money that I had saved during the year, but I was determined to see some of the world. We bought a round-the-world ticket, which included flights to Thailand, Malaysia, Indonesia, Australia, New Zealand and America, with lots of overland travel in between. The trip was fantastic and really allowed us to experience different cultures and ways of life. It also provided a sense of freedom, which I never dreamt of whilst at school or working. The opportunities to scuba dive, go jungle trekking and sail were fantastic and will remain with me for the rest of my life.

Overall, I thoroughly enjoyed my year out and would recommend that everyone take one. Although medicine is a long course, the skills that can be learnt in a year out can be invaluable to potential doctors.

Chapter 5 **Choosing a medical school**

5.1 So many to choose from

In 1997 approximately 12 000 people applied to study medicine at 27 medical schools in the UK and just over 5000 were accepted. Following this there was a small but gradual decline in applications until 2002. Since then there has been a dramatic increase in applicants and although more places at medical school the competition is now greater. The opening of several new medical schools in the last few years has increased the number of institutions offering a medical degree to thirty-one. The table below summarises the changes in applicant to acceptance ratio for the last few years (Source: UCAS 2006).

Year	Number of applicants	Number accepted
2005	19 360	7821
2004	17 826	7955
2003	14 833	7667
2002	11 935	6959
2001	10 231	6240
2000	10 226	5714
1999	10 972	5312
1998	11 807	5119
1997	12 076	5029
1996	12 025	4894

Some medical schools receive over 3000 applications each year. These figures include overseas applicants, who account for around 10% of all undergraduate medical students accepted on courses. Chapter 2 gave advice concerning the medical school application procedure, but the next real question is, 'Which universities should I apply to?' There is a vast array of medical schools, each with individual characteristics and idiosyncrasies yet, paradoxically, from an initial inspection of the UCAS handbook, all the universities appear to be too similar to differentiate. This chapter will help guide you through the selection process, demonstrating that, when various criteria are applied, there are significant differences between them, which will help you decide which ones are right for you.

5.2 Does it really matter which one I choose?

From a superficial view point it doesn't really matter which medical school you attend because at the end of the course you will graduate with a degree that will allow you to practise as a medical doctor (do not get confused by the fact different establishments offer varying qualifications i.e. MB, ChB, BM). That aside, there are many reasons to take time over deciding where to apply because the universities can vary considerably – location, type of school, reputation, quality of teaching, format of curriculum, assessments, availability of an intercalated degree and more. Whilst some of these factors may not be important to you, others will.

5.3 How should I go about choosing a medical school?

For applications in 2007, there are 5 medical schools in London (a few years ago there were many more than this but there have been several mergers and they are now all affiliated to the University of London) and 24 universities outside London that have departments of medicine. Oxford and Cambridge universities also offer degrees in medicine. This makes a total of 31 institutions which offer undergraduate medical courses.

The UCAS form asks candidates to list six choices of course and establishment. As discussed in Chapter 2, only four of these choices can be medical courses. You should seek advice from your school or college on whether to

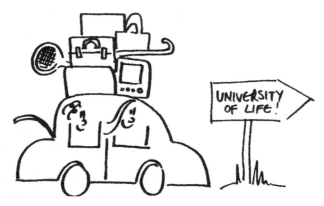

University of life

complete the other two slots with an alternative type of course, or leave it blank. Contrary to popular belief, the universities DO NOT know which other establishments you have applied to until the offers have already been made. However they can see if you have applied to more than one course at that individual university.

Medical school choices

- University of Aberdeen
- University of Birmingham
- Brighton and Sussex Medical School
- University of Bristol
- University of Cambridge
- Cardiff University
- University of Dundee
- University of East Anglia (Norwich)
- University of Edinburgh
- University of Glasgow
- Hull and York Medical School
- University of Keele (= Manchester degree)
- University of Leeds
- University of Leicester
- University of Liverpool
- University of Manchester
- University of Newcastle-upon-Tyne
- University of Nottingham
- University of Oxford
- Peninsula Medical School (Exeter and Plymouth)
- Queens University Belfast
- University of Sheffield
- University of Southampton
- University of St. Andrews
- University of Wales Swansea
- University of Warwick

London University Medical Schools

- Imperial College, London
- Kings College, London
- Queen Mary, University of London
- St George's, University of London
- University College London

Things to consider before making a choice on the UCAS form are:
* Competition for places
* Cost of living in the area
* How easy it is to find accommodation as a student
* Style of teaching on the course
* Assessment methods
* Degree of community-based teaching
* Balance between theory and practise
* Facilities – both academic and social
* Life in and around the university town
* Whether you want to mix with students outside medicine
* Whether you are likely to get the high grades needed to be offered a place in a medical school.

5.4 The factors

Academic reputation

Although mentioned first, it is not the most important factor. Whilst for many subjects, students would be advised to attend the most prestigious university possible; in medicine it is a little different. Whereas Oxbridge is the pinnacle in most subject areas, they offer a different approach to medical education, which will not necessarily suit everybody. Years ago, there was a certain degree of elitism amongst some medical schools, but the tide seems to have turned with more pioneering medical schools now enjoying a certain degree of elitism themselves, proclaiming that they produce doctors better equipped to deal with medicine in the 21st century. Purely academic candidates do not always make the best doctors. One should consider the medical school's syllabus rather than its reputation.

Traditionally medical students were placed in a lecture theatre for 2 years and then allowed on the wards for the next 3 years. Most medical schools have designed modern curricula introducing an integrated approach and embracing ward-based teaching much earlier on. Places with high academic reputations will be keen to maintain them and are likely to work their students harder, but this does not guarantee that they produce better doctors.

University or medical school?

Universities have the advantage of a large campus, with students studying a variety of other, non-medical, subjects. Most students prefer the mixing of medical and non-medical students during the early years as, during the pure clinical years, it is inevitable that more time will be spent with just medical students. This is mainly due to the combination of other students having a shorter course and medics having little in the way of holiday in the later years. Pure medical schools mean that you will be socialising mainly with medical students, but this could mean a closer knit community.

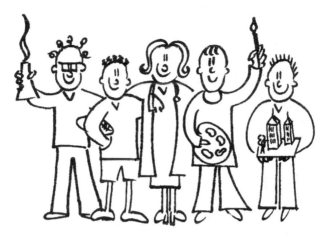

Universities have the advantage of students studying a variety of other, non-medical subjects

Career Intentions

Only rarely do medical school applicants know which speciality they wish to pursue. There are, however, particular places and hospitals in the country that specialise in a particular aspect of a subject. For example:
- Spinal surgery – Stoke Mandeville
- Trauma – Birmingham
- Eyes – Moorfields
- Children – Great Ormond Street.

If you had a true insight into your career intentions, you might consider going to a particular place that will allow you to indulge your career fantasies. We do not think this should influence your decision as the majority of newly qualified doctors often change their career decision following graduation.

Type of course

Aren't they all the same?

Whilst everybody qualifies as a doctor at the end (provided you have passed!), there are significant differences between the courses. The basic course design is essentially the same, as the medical curriculum is partly dictated from a national body. There have been major changes in course content, methods of teaching and assessment processes over the last 10 years. These have in part been led by the General Medical Council's recommendations for the future training of medical students.

Integrated versus traditional
The traditional method of teaching medicine was to have medical school based lectures and tutorials for the first 2–3 years and then students would don a white coat, buy a stethoscope and be taught on the hospital wards until graduation. Most medical schools now take a more integrated method and combine these two, previously dichotomous approaches. In theory, this familiarises students more quickly and allows them to see the clinical relevance of the theory that they are learning in the lecture theatre. There are only a minority of medical schools that keep to the more traditional methods and these often have a 3-year preclinical course which includes a higher degree (e.g. Oxbridge and St. Andrews).

Course length
For most establishments the course is 5 years. If the preclinical course is a full 3 years (see above), then this increases to 6 years. This is also the case if a student enrols on a foundation medicine course. Graduate entry courses are 4 years and this is due to shorter holidays and slightly compacted curricula. As financial restraints are sometimes a problem, course length could certainly be a factor when deciding upon choice of medical school.

Extra degree
At most universities there is an option of taking a further year to undertake an extra degree. At some medical schools this is an integral part of the course. This involves a period of research or lecture-based course, and will culminate in a degree such as a BSc or MA. This degree can certainly be a useful addition to your curriculum vitae when applying for jobs. It also allows students to take a short break from medicine or indulge a particular research interest. It is sometimes possible to continue the degree into a PhD which will take a further 2 years. One other advantage is that if at this stage a student does not feel they wish to continue to the clinical years, they can leave university with an alternative degree.

Town or country?
Medical schools are usually located within major towns or cities, but some are more rural in location. This might have a bearing if you wish to

pursue or take up a particular sport or activity. The surfing is not great in Birmingham!

Proximity to home

This is always a frequently mentioned factor when people are initially making a decision about their choice of medical school. The prospect of leaving parents, a partner or rugby team can certainly be too much for some, and they choose the nearest medical school. Whilst this should not be considered to be a mistake, one of the benefits of leaving for university is to gain independence. Living in the same town as your parents and friends can stifle this ability. If you really do not wish to leave your parents too far behind, choose a university that is only a short journey away.

There are a huge number of reasons why a student might want or need to stay near their family. If your only motivation is that you might miss them and it would be convenient to pop home once in a while, we might suggest that you should go a little further afield. Regular trips home to allow your mother to iron your T-shirts may impair your integration into medical school and university life. In some circumstances it may be necessary from a financial perspective to stay near home or even live with loved ones. Again we would advise to think carefully before committing.

Cost of travel

Whilst we might advocate not living in the same city as your parents, you will probably want to return home during term time. The further away from home, the greater the cost of travel. If travelling from Scotland to Plymouth, these costs could be significant.

Future career location

This is a relatively commonly cited reason for choosing a medical school in a particular part of the country. Whilst some doctors stay in the place they studied, this is infrequent and most doctors move around the country before deciding where to practise long term. Frequently, with the best jobs being very competitive, moving is forced rather than optional. Location can become increasingly important as you climb the career ladder.

Accommodation

The quality and level of provision of accommodation by medical schools varies significantly, although most universities do guarantee first year students some accommodation. Some cities have plentiful cheap accommodation close to the university but rent can vary considerably, and, as medicine is a 5-year course, the cumulative cost can be significant. The relative lack of accommo-dation available in and around London means extra expense, considerable commuting times and less value for money. Whilst this is not a good enough reason to justify going to one university over another, it is certainly worth bearing in mind. More of this subject is covered in Chapter 9.

Gap year

This subject is covered in Chapter 4, but it is worth bearing in mind that some medical schools can look more favourably upon a gap year than others. If you take a gap year, you may want to be with other people who have also taken a gap year.

Strategic applications

Your decision on which medical school to attend should be a personal one. After all you are going to spend up to 6 years of your life there. It is worth noting, however, that some medical schools are more popular than others, and if you apply only to these, you might reduce your chance of a successful application. Most doctors we know confess to having made a spread bet appli-cation, applying to some popular and some less popular schools. It is also worth applying to institutions that offer different entry requirements, in case your A level results are lower than expected.

What about my other interests?

Inevitably, you will want to know which medical schools cater for your partic-ular extracurricular activities. It is likely that most universities will be able to cater for you, but check this before you go. Whilst medical school is fairly demanding, there is some opportunity for other hobbies and, with a little time management, you can keep several activities going.

5.5 Other options – private medical schools

For students who may be struggling to gain a place at medical school or who realise their A level results may not be sufficient for entry into one of the uni-versities mentioned above, there are now some other options. There are a growing number of the so-called private medical schools that accept applica-tions from British school leavers. Despite many of these courses being located in foreign countries, the curriculum is taught in English. Some examples include St Charles University in Prague, St Matthews University in the Cayman Islands and St Georges in the Caribbean. There are also some courses (e.g. School of Health and Neural Sciences, Nottingham), that have courses run in the UK using foreign curriculae (usually US). If the course is a US based 4-year degree then it would be necessary to complete a pre-med year at one of the courses in the UK. The main disadvantages to these courses are the cost and the fact that it is often necessary to sit further exams if a trainee wishes to return to the UK to work (a graduate would be classed as an overseas trainee). The main advantage is that these courses often accept lower entry requirements (e.g. BBC). We would recommend researching about these options very carefully before applying. One website worth a look is www.readmedicine.co.uk.

5.6 Summary

A common theme when you visit universities is that the students who show you around will try and persuade you that their medical school is the best in the country (if they don't then it is probably worth avoiding!). When looking around the university, time is probably spent more profitably chatting to current students and looking around the university campus at accommodation and bars etc. Having a guided tour of a medical school is less useful because the facilities will be similar between institutions (see Chapter 9). It is essential that you talk to as many students as possible to get a feel for the real situation including both the academic and social arrangements. The information included in this chapter can certainly help to cut down your choice of medical school, but at the end of the day if you have a gut feeling, go with it. The odds are that you will have a brilliant time at whichever institution you end up attending.

The best way to find your future medical school is to . . .
- GO THERE!
- Attend the open days
- Meet people
- Talk to current/ex-students
- Talk to staff
- Read the prospectus and alternative prospectus
- Look around the town
- Check out the websites mentioned in the appendix

University	GCE entry requirements	A levels	AS levels	Other qualifications considered	Graduate entry?	Pre-medical/ access course?
Aberdeen	AAB	Acceptable on its own and combined with other qualifications. Chemistry is highly desirable, plus at least one from Biology, Mathematics or Physics and one other. General Studies excluded.	Acceptable only when combined with other qualifications. General Studies excluded.			
Barts, London, Queen Mary	AAB	Acceptable on its own and combined with other qualifications. Chemistry or Biology. General Studies excluded.	Acceptable combined with other qualifications. Biology at grade B and Chemistry at grade B required. General Studies excluded.	ASVCE, AVCE, AVCE Double Award not acceptable.	Available	
Birmingham	AAB	Acceptable on its own and combined with other qualifications. Chemistry and either Biology or Physics or Mathematics. Human Biology may be offered, but not in addition to Biology. General Studies excluded.	Acceptable only when combined with other qualifications. Biology at AS level is required if not offered at A level. Human Biology may be offered instead of Biology.	ASVCE, AVCE, AVCE Double Awards, FSMQ and AEA acceptable only when combined with other qualifications.	Available	
Brighton and Sussex	340 tariff points	Acceptable on its own and combined with other	Acceptable combined with other qualifications. Chemistry	ASVCE, AVCE, AEA, AVCE Double		

	qualifications. Biology or Chemistry required. General Studies excluded.	and Biology. General Studies excluded.	Awards – Acceptable combined with other qualifications. AVCE and AVCE Double Awards – Science required.		Available
Bristol	AAB	Acceptable on its own and combined with other qualifications. Chemistry at grade A required. General Studies excluded.	Acceptable combined with other qualifications. If four AS levels offered at least one should be in a non-science subject.	ASVCE, AVCE, AVCE Double Award, BTEC National Award acceptable only when combined with other qualifications.	Available Available
Cambridge	AAA	Acceptable on its own and combined with other qualifications. One from Biology, Chemistry, Physics or Mathematics. Chemistry required at least to AS level.	Acceptable only when combined with other qualifications. Three of Biology, Chemistry, Physics, Mathematics.	FSMQ and AEA acceptable only when combined with other subjects.	Available
Cardiff	370 tariff points	Acceptable on its own and combined with other qualifications. Two of Chemistry, Biology, Physics, Mathematics, Statistics.	Acceptable only when combined with other qualifications. Chemistry or Biology if not taken at A Level at grade B. General Studies excluded.	ASVCE and AVCE acceptable only when combined with other qualifications. Health and Social Care preferred.	Available
Dundee	AAA	Acceptable on its own and combined with other qualifications. Chemistry and any science subject at grade A. General Studies excluded.	Not acceptable.		Available

(Continued)

(Continued)

University	GCE entry requirements	A levels	AS levels	Other qualifications considered	Graduate entry?	Pre-medical/access course?
East Anglia	AAB	Acceptable on its own and combined with other qualifications. Biology should be at least at B grade. General Studies excluded.	Acceptable only when combined with other qualifications.	ASVCE, AVCE, AVCE Double Award, FSMQ and AEA acceptable only when combined with other subjects. For AVCE and AVCE Double Awards, Health and Social Sciences preferred.		
Edinburgh	AAAb	Acceptable on its own and combined with other qualifications. Chemistry and any of Mathematics, Physics or Biology.	Acceptable only when combined with other qualifications. Biology required if not held at A level.	ASVCE and AVCE acceptable only when combined with other subjects.		Available
Glasgow	AAB	Acceptable on its own and combined with other qualifications. Chemistry required and one from Biology, Mathematics or Physics. Biology or Human Biology in addition to Chemistry is preferred.				

				Available	Available
Guy's, King's and St Thomas', London	AABc	Acceptable on its own and combined with other qualifications. Biology at grade B or Chemistry at grade B required. General Studies excluded.	Acceptable only when combined with other qualifications. General Studies excluded.	ASVCE, AEA and Welsh Baccalaureate acceptable only when combined with other subjects.	
Hull York	AABb	Acceptable on its own and combined with other qualifications. Chemistry and Biology required. General Studies excluded.	Acceptable only when combined with other qualifications. Biology and Chemistry required.	ASVCE, AVCE acceptable only when combined with other subjects.	
Imperial College, London	AABb	Acceptable on its own and combined with other qualifications. Biology or Chemistry required. General Studies excluded.	Acceptable combined with other qualifications. Biology and Chemistry required. General Studies excluded.	ASVCE, AVCE, AVCE Double Award not acceptable.	
Keele	AAB	Grades AAB required from Chemistry plus either Biology/ Physics/Maths plus one further academic subject if only two sciences are offered.	Not acceptable.	ASVCE, AVCE, AVCE Double Award not acceptable.	
Leeds	AAB	Acceptable on its own and combined with other qualifications. Chemistry required. General Studies excluded.	Acceptable only when combined with other qualifications.	ASVCE, AVCE, AVCE Double Award acceptable only when combined with other subjects.	

(Continued)

(Continued)

University	GCE entry requirements	A levels	AS levels	Other qualifications considered	Graduate entry?	Pre-medical/access course?
Leicester	AAB	Acceptable on its own and combined with other qualifications. Chemistry required at grade A. General Studies excluded.	Acceptable combined with other qualifications. Biology and Chemistry required. General Studies excluded.	ASVCE, AVCE, AVCE Double Award, FSMQ and AEA acceptable only when combined with other subjects.	Available	
Liverpool	AAB	Acceptable on its own and combined with other qualifications. Chemistry required at grade A.	Acceptable combined with other qualifications. Biology and Chemistry required. General Studies acceptable.	ASVCE, AVCE, AVCE Double Award, FSMQ and AEA acceptable only when combined with other subjects.	Available	
Manchester	AAB	Acceptable on its own and combined with other qualifications. Chemistry and one other of Biology, Physics, Human Biology or Mathematics. General Studies excluded.	Acceptable only when combined with other qualifications. General Studies excluded.	ASVCE, AVCE, AVCE Double Award, FSMQ, AEA and BTEC National Award acceptable only when combined with other qualifications.		Available
Newcastle	AAA	Acceptable on its own and combined with other qualifications. Chemistry or Biology required. General Studies excluded.	Acceptable only when combined with other qualifications.	ASVCE, AVCE, AVCE. Double Award, AEA and BTEC National Award acceptable only when combined with other qualifications	Available	

Nottingham	AAB	Acceptable on its own and combined with other qualifications. Chemistry and Biology (or Human Biology) at A grade. General Studies excluded.	Acceptable only when combined with other qualifications.	Welsh Baccalaureate acceptable combined with other qualifications.	Available
Oxford	AAA	Acceptable on its own and combined with other qualifications. Chemistry with either Mathematics or Biology or Physics.	Acceptable only when combined with other qualifications. General Studies excluded.	ASVCE, AVCE, AVCE Double Award, FSMQ, AEA and BTEC National Award acceptable only when combined with other qualifications. Welsh Baccalaureate acceptable combined with other qualifications.	Available
Peninsula	370 tariff points	Acceptable on its own and combined with other qualifications. Biology or Chemistry or Mathematics or Physics plus two further subjects at A level, preferably to include one non-science subject.	Acceptable combined with other qualifications. General Studies excluded.	ASVCE, AVCE, AVCE Double Award, FSMQ, AEA and BTEC National Award acceptable only when combined with other qualifications. Welsh Baccalaureate acceptable combined with other qualifications.	

(Continued)

(*Continued.*)

University	GCE entry requirements	A levels	AS levels	Other qualifications considered	Graduate entry?	Pre-medical/access course?
Queens University, Belfast	AAAa	Acceptable only when combined with other qualifications. Chemistry at grade A and (Biology at grade A or Mathematics at grade A or Physics at grade A). General Studies excluded.	Acceptable only when combined with other qualifications. General Studies excluded.	ASCVE, AVCE, AVCE Double Award acceptable combined with other subjects.		
Sheffield	AAB	Acceptable on its own and combined with other qualifications. Chemistry and any Science subject.	Acceptable only when combined with other qualifications. Chemistry, Biology and one other science subject recommended.	ASVCE not acceptable. AVCE acceptable combined with other subjects.		Available
Southampton	AAB	Acceptable on its own and combined with other qualifications. Chemistry required.	Acceptable only when combined with other qualifications.	ASVCE, AVCE, AVCE Double Award and BTEC National Award acceptable combined with other qualifications.	Available	
St Andrews	AAB	Acceptable on its own and combined with other qualifications. Chemistry and	Acceptable only when combined with other qualifications.			

Biology. Mathematics or Physics. General Studies excluded.

St George's, London	AABb–BBCb	Acceptable on its own and combined with other qualifications. Chemistry and Biology required. General Studies excluded.	Not acceptable.	ASVCE, AVCE, AVCE Double Award not acceptable. AEA and Welsh Baccalaureate acceptable combined with other qualifications.	Available
Swansea	Graduate entry course	Partnership arrangement with Cardiff for 5 year medical degree. Contact medical school for further details.			Available
University College London	AABe	Acceptable on its own and combined with other qualifications. Chemistry and biology required.	Acceptable only when combined with other qualifications.	ASVCE, AVCE, AVCE Double Award – Acceptable combined with other qualifications.	
Warwick	Graduate entry course	Candidates are expected to have a first class or good upper second class degree in Biological Sciences. Relevant work experience is essential.			Available

AEA: Advanced Extension Awards; ASVCE: Advanced Subsidiary Vocational Certificate of Education; AVCE: Advanced Vocational Certificate in Education; BTEC: Business and Technology Education Council; FSMQ: Free Standing Maths Qualification; GCE: General Certificate of Education.

PERSONAL VIEW *Zudin Puthucheary*

I am a Malaysian citizen but spent the latter part of my school life and university time in the UK. Since graduation in 1997, I have worked for the NHS apart from a 3-year break in Australia. Times have changed for overseas medical students and if you aim to work here post-qualification you must clarify the possibilities of working as a doctor in this country *before* entering medical school. Recently there have been some important changes to work permits for non-UK nationals. Additionally, in many countries more medical schools are being set up, especially in South East Asia. Check that the qualifications you hope to gain in this country will be recognised on your return home. Clarify if you will be required to work in a supervised fashion back in your country of residency and if local graduates will have 'better' jobs earmarked for them. This form of protectionism does exist around the world in medicine, regardless of the quality of your training. Aside from your degree, some countries will expect you to sit further exams on your return, to qualify for unrestricted registration with their Medical Council. In short, think carefully about your long term plan – if your ultimate goal is to work in your home country but you consider the education system 'superior' in the UK, make sure this will not be frowned upon.

Financial planning is desperately important, especially if you are not studying on a scholarship. Your credit rating will be non-existent, and student life can be hard in this situation when it comes to renting accommodation, hiring cars and applying for credit cards. If you know several years in advance that you're planning to study here, open a bank account at that stage, and if you are self-funded, have your parents do so as well. Regular payments into this account are better than a lump sum for your credit rating. It may help to get a letter of 'good credit' or a reference from your local bank.

A lasting comment from a friend of mine from Malaysia, who also happened to be one of my seniors was, 'are you going to dress like a foreigner, or like a Brit?' His feeling was that there is always a large expat community at medical school, but to really get the best out of my time, he thought I should learn to integrate. The culture shock is often overwhelming and it is natural to turn to your fellow countrymen due to often common interests. However, to overcome this properly, takes time and interaction with the locals. I'm told that anthropologists feel at least a year is necessary to understand a different culture! Over the years, whilst keeping in contact with the Malaysian and Singaporean Society, I made good friends with the British members of my year and enjoyed my time tremendously. Having a strong support network among my friends and colleagues is even more important with my family so far away. Following university I decided

(Continued)

(*Continued.*)

to remain in the UK and complete some of my early professional training as the training and exam structure in the UK is internationally recognised.

That racism is rife in the NHS is agreed – there have been several publications on this nature. It wasn't until recently I grasped the ideology behind the institutional racism. I was in Sydney talking to the Australian registrar I was dating, when she told me she really had little time for non-Australians doctors or patients especially those who didn't speak good English. It struck me that while at work she couldn't see past the cufflinks, Saville row shirt or the (now) British accent, to my skin colour. The NHS employs 1 million people. People are people, good or bad. Racism is not about colour these days, it is about being different, and my European colleagues working in the UK have similar stories despite the UK being increasingly cosmopolitan. My first experience of racism was in clinic when a patient refused to shake 'the darkie's' hand in the waiting room. I dealt with this case calmly and professionally, and every other patient who walked into my consulting room apologised profusely, hoping I didn't believe they were all like that.

So why train here? In my opinion the medical school training here is world class, and the integrated, problem based teaching programmes now seen world wide take many of there origins from the UK. On a personal level, living in a different country gives you a new perspective on life, and a chance to see very different attitudes, and to overcome your own preconceived views. My advice is to attempt to integrate as much as possible without forgetting your roots. You are living in a foreign country, and you don't really know what your future holds (I've been here for 14 years, still occasionally wondering about going home, mostly during winter!). Medicine is an institution, and you can make great friends, regardless of race, religion or colour. Your friends are also your coping mechanisms, which you will need at more difficult times.

Chapter 6 Applying to Oxbridge

This chapter has been added, not because Oxford and Cambridge are better than other medical schools but because they have very different courses, application procedures, and rules and regulations. This can make the whole process pretty confusing.

6.1 The basic facts

First of all, you can only apply to *either* Cambridge or Oxford and not both (unless you want to be an Organ Scholar!). Both Oxford and Cambridge Universities are composed of about 30 colleges each. Currently each college interviews its own applicants and awards places at that particular college within the university. This means that you will become a member of a particular college at the university (for example, St John's College, Cambridge). The total number of medical students is split between the colleges. Not all colleges take the same number of students and the number at any one college varies from about 3 to around 26!

6.2 The differences in the course

Cambridge and Oxford both have quite traditional courses. Students undertake 3 years of undergraduate study before they go to the hospital and start the clinical course. The first 2 years have a compulsory syllabus which covers the basic sciences. In year 3 you undertake a compulsory intercalated degree that leads to the BA (Bachelor of Arts) degree. Oxbridge does not award BSc (Bachelor of Science) degrees for historical reasons. Bizarrely, also for historical reasons, this degree becomes automatically converted to an MA (Master of Arts) about 3 years after you finish your BA!

There are some differences specific to Cambridge. There is an examination system called the Tripos system. The first year exams are called part 1a, the second year exams are called part 1b, and the third year exams are called part 2. Each year is graded using the usual degree classes, that is 1st, 2:1, 2:2 and 3rd. If you get a first in part 1 (average of part 1a and 1b) and part 2 then you get the famous double first. This is extremely uncommon! Otherwise, the third year grade is the final degree that you get. If you get a 2:2 (or better) in the Cambridge exams in the first and second years then you automatically also pass the professional medical exams (second MB) in that subject and can proceed to the next lot of exams!

In Oxford the first and second year exams for each subject are graded: distinction (rare), pass or fail. In the third year they are graded according to the traditional degree grades (1st, 2:1, 2:2, 3rd), and this is the degree you end up with from Oxford.

6.3 The colleges

Currently, the individual colleges are responsible for interviewing you and offering a place. Not all of the colleges accept undergraduate medical students; check which ones take medical students, how many they accept each year and find out how many applicants they received in the preceding year.

The college provides accommodation, dining and most other living facilities (for example, bar, gym, boat club, tennis courts, squash courts, playing fields, music rooms, etc.). The college has a mix of students from all different subjects. Each of the colleges has its own societies: sports teams, orchestras, drama groups, discussion groups, religious groups, etc. The colleges within the university compete against each other in most of the sports and most famously in rowing. In addition to this side of college life, the colleges organise small group teaching (tutorials or supervisions) with often only two, three or four students. These are with a specialist tutor linked to that particular college. This small group teaching is individual to the college and in addition to other teaching organised by the University. This style of teaching is unique to Oxbridge.

Choosing a college is difficult. The first thing to do is to look at the college prospectuses either online at:
- http://www.cam.ac.uk/admissions/undergraduate (Cambridge)
- http://www.admissions.ox.ac.uk (Oxford)

or obtain a paper copy of the university prospectus:
- fill in an online application at:
  http://www.cam.ac.uk/admissions/undergraduate/publications/prospectus.html (Cambridge)
- email:
  undergraduate.admissions@admin.ox.ac.uk (Oxford) and give your name and address.

This will give you basic information about each college. Look at the number of students they take per year and how many applicants they had for medicine last year. The best way is to visit those you are interested in and form your own opinions. The average number of applicants per place in 2005 at Oxford was 7 per place across all the colleges. Each college has its own atmosphere and, if you feel you fit in, then it is more likely that the people interviewing you will feel that as well! Go to the open days (see the prospectus for details) and see what they say, but also visit independently and browse around the colleges. Speak to the students there and find out as much as possible. It looks good in interview if you can show that you have made the effort and found out as much as possible.

Traditionally in Cambridge, Gonville & Caius (pronounced *keys*), and Downing College have large numbers of medical students every year and the old and famous colleges such as King's, Trinity and St John's are always popular. There are currently about 280 students per year at Cambridge studying medicine. Oxford has far fewer medical students in each year (about 150) and there are no really big medical colleges. Most have about four to six students. The very wealthy old colleges in Oxford are Magdalen (pronounced *maw-de-len*), Christchurch, St John's and New College.

6.4 The universities

There are no medical departments at Oxford or Cambridge. Each of the undergraduate subjects (for example, anatomy, biochemistry, physiology, etc.) has its own department within the university and students from all the colleges will meet for lectures and practical classes organised by these departments. All medical students will therefore get the same lectures and practical classes, but the small group teaching organised by the colleges will be different depending on which college you attend.

Work aside, all the social activities available at college level are also represented at a university level. This means that selection for the university teams is from students from all the colleges. Traditionally medical students have been well represented in university sports including rugby, rowing, etc. If you represent your university at sport you may receive the famous blue: light blue for Cambridge and dark blue for Oxford. The famous annual Oxford–Cambridge boat race on the Thames and the Oxford varsity rugby match attract avid support every year.

6.5 The application process

The first step in the application process is to register for the BMAT (Bio-Medical Admissions Test) exam (see Chapter 3). The deadline for BMAT registration is the end of September. You will need a BMAT registration number to put on your application forms.

The next step is to complete your UCAS (University and Colleges Admission Service) form and either the Cambridge application form (CAF) or the Oxford application form (OAF).

The CAF is at: http://www.cam.ac.uk/admissions/undergraduate/ apply/
                   forms/undergraduate.pdf
The OAF is at: http://www.admissions.ox.ac.uk/forms

If you apply to Oxbridge you must list *either* Oxford or Cambridge as one of your choices on your UCAS form. The UCAS and Cambridge/Oxford application form must be received before the middle of October the year before you want to start your course. Copies of the application forms should be available through your school. You can either choose one college from the list of those accepting undergraduates or you can put an open application, which means the university will allocate you to a college.

In Oxford, the last women-only college has recently voted (June 2006) to admit men in the coming years. Although when this will take effect has yet to be decided. There are numerous graduate/mature student colleges in Oxford that do not accept medical undergraduates. This is made clear in the advice sheet that accompanies the application form.

In Cambridge, Newnham and New Hall are for women only. There are several colleges that are primarily for postgraduate students (for example, those doing PhDs), which accept a few mature students (that is those over 21) to do undergraduate subjects. These include Wolfson, Hugh's Hall and Lucy Cavendish (women over 21 only). Homerton does not currently accept medical students.

After you have submitted your UCAS and OAF/CAF form, the next step in the application process is the BMAT test. This is at the beginning of November and is normally taken in your school/college. The results will be available for the universities at the end of November. Interviews will then take place in December.

6.6 The selection procedure

To get a place at Oxbridge, it is almost assumed you will get at least three A grades at 'A' level (or equivalent). The entrance process is constantly evolving and further changes are anticipated in the next few years. At present all applicants must take the BMAT. It is the responsibility of candidates to ensure they are registered for BMAT (see www.bmat.org.uk for information on how to register). You must register to take the BMAT if you want to apply to Cambridge,

Table 6.1 Timetable for applications

Date	Oxbridge application process
Mid-September	Closing date for requests for special versions of BMAT question papers (Braille or enlarged text)
End September	Standard closing date for BMAT test
Mid-October	Late entry for BMAT closing date (subject to penalty fees)
Mid-October	Closing date for UCAS and OAF/CUF forms
Beginning November	BMAT test date
Early to mid-December	Interviews
End December to Early January	Results

Note: Check the websites for the exact dates which alter slightly from year to year.

Oxford, University College London or Imperial College London. Applications from candidates who have not registered to take the BMAT test will not be considered.

Shortlisting for interview will be based on previous academic (GCSE, General Certificate of Secondary Education) performance, BMAT score and other information provided in your UCAS application. In Oxford about one-third of applicants will be invited to interview at two different colleges. One of the colleges will be the college of first choice (or assignment if an open application has been made), the second college will be randomly assigned. You will be required to spend a night or two in Oxford in mid-December in order to attend the interviews. In Cambridge you will be interviewed in early to mid-December by your first choice college (or assigned college if an open application has been made) if your application is successful. No places will be awarded without interview.

6.7 Interviews

First read the interview chapter (Chapter 6) for general advice in this area. The Oxbridge interviews are held in December and have a reputation for being crazy and difficult. You will hear all sorts of stories about being thrown rugby balls and seeing what you do, or being ignored until you say something – these are untrue. Most colleges have two interviews. There tends to be a medical suitability interview with clinically practising doctors and then an academic suitability interview with the college academics. This is designed to see if you are academically strong enough and will fit in with the tutorial style, academic course, etc. In the academic interview you may be asked strange questions to which you don't know the answers. This is intentional. They are trying to see what you can do on the spot under the pressure of an interview and what you can work out for yourself.

Stay calm, be yourself, listen to the question carefully, think before you say anything stupid and then have a go at the question. You should not be easily led from your opinion if you really think that you are right but should be flexible and not so rigid that you can't accept other ideas. They are looking to see that you can argue a point and contribute to a discussion. Finally, be prepared to say 'I don't know' if you are really stuck! The interviews usually last about 20 minutes.

6.8 Offers

Like all other universities you will be made a conditional offer. This is usually for three grade As in your A levels. You will be notified by post and it usually arrives around Christmas time. Traditionally Oxford notifies applicants just before Christmas and Cambridge just after!

Occasionally some candidates are considered by other colleges in what is known as the 'pool'. This is a complicated system in which good candidates are offered places at other colleges if the colleges have not managed to find students of adequate standard from their own applicants. This process may delay your offer and may occasionally require another interview.

6.9 Rejection

If you don't get in, try not to despair as you still have two options. Firstly, you can go to one of your other UCAS choices if you are made an offer. You have not failed and will have a fantastic time somewhere else. Secondly, you can take a gap year and reapply the following year. If you applied to Oxford the first time round, you may try Cambridge the next year and vice versa, or you may try applying to a different college at the same university the second time round! Bear in mind that you must achieve a minimum of three grade As at A level to make it worth reapplying.

If you don't get your necessary grades

If you have an offer but then miss your required grades by a small margin it is worth getting in touch with the college and speaking to the medical tutor for that college. Explain your situation and see if they will still consider taking you. It is worth a try but they may still reject you.

6.10 Conclusion

Oxford and Cambridge are internationally renowned institutions and this results in steep competition for places. All the candidates have very good grades at GCSE/AS level and are predicted to do well at A level. The courses are more academic and the teaching is generally more traditional in style. The college system can make things a bit confusing at first and there is the hassle of a different application form and entrance exam. However, Oxford and Cambridge are unique and fantastic places to study medicine. Have a go – it is worth a try!

6.11 Useful information

Cambridge
- General information about the university: http://www.cam.ac.uk
- Applying for medicine: http://www.cam.ac.uk/admissions/undergraduate/
- Address for obtaining university prospectus:

CAO, Kellet Lodge, Tennis Court Road, Cambridge, CB2 1QJ
Telephone: +44 (0) 1223 333308

Oxford
- General information about the university: http://www.ox.ac.uk
- About the course: http://www.admissions.ox.ac.uk/courses/medi.shtml
- Address for obtaining university prospectus:

Admissions Information Centre, 67 St Giles, Oxford

Chapter 7 **The interview process**

Interviews are the part of the application process that most students dread. The idea of being sat in front of a panel of doctors and/or academics, and being asked to justify why you think you are good enough to be studying medicine at their medical school is daunting. The vast majority of medical schools interview their applicants. Currently, those that do not interview are Aberdeen, Belfast, Edinburgh, Southampton and St Andrew's.

Things to remember:

- You will spend many years at the medical school you attend, so you need to be sure that it is the right place for you. You must choose them as much as them choosing you!
- For UK applicants in 2005 there were 2.5 applicants per medical school place. That's not bad odds!
- Make sure that you prepare as much as possible.

7.1 Preparation

Preparation is the key to success. You need to think about whether you want to go to medical school and which one will suit you, as early as possible. Go and visit the medical schools, formulate your opinions and see if you think you would fit in. Once you are sure that you want to become a doctor, you will need to work on things to put in your personal statement on your UCAS form. This is, in effect, your CV and is your opportunity to sell yourself. The interviewers are not looking for someone who is just academically good; they want students who are well rounded individuals with a variety of interests. Spend time on your personal statement and get other people (parents/teachers) to read and check it. Occasionally candidates get carried away and in their enthusiasm to impress they exaggerate and start to make up extra bits. Don't be tempted to do this because, if you are found out, your credibility is ruined and you will not get a place.

7.2 While you are waiting

Once your UCAS form is sent off there will be a considerable time (usually months) before you go for interview. Make sure that you keep a copy of your UCAS form so that you can remind yourself about what you wrote before the interview. Use the time between sending off your UCAS form and the interviews to practise what you are going to say. Get your teachers/parents/friends to arrange mock interviews. Take this seriously and listen to the feedback that the interviewers provide. You can improve your interview style and answers with practise. It will feel more natural on the day, and will often mean that you have formulated the answers and heard them out loud before the real thing. You can also practice on your own by asking yourself a simple, straightforward question like, 'Why do you want to be a doctor?' and then answering out loud. The first time it will seem strange and you will make a real mess of the answer, but after a couple of goes it becomes more natural.

7.3 On the day of the interview

You will receive a request for interview by post from the medical schools. This will outline where and when your interview(s) will take place. Hopefully you will have visited the medical school before so you will know roughly where you are going. Allow plenty of time to get to your interview, travel the night before if necessary. If you miss your appointment time you may not be offered an alternative.

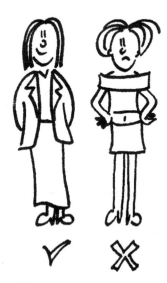

At interview . . . dress to look like a doctor

What to wear

The advice in the letter from the medical school usually says something like 'Wear what you feel comfortable in'. This is standard advice for applicants of all subjects. However, you are applying to be a doctor, and will be interviewed by doctors and consequently are expected to project the image of a doctor. Why make things awkward? It is better to be too smart than underdressed. You will feel more confident if you are smart, and are less likely to feel uncomfortable or embarrassed.

Men could wear a shirt and tie, with smart trousers and a jacket, or a plain suit, with polished shoes. It is more difficult to be specific about women but either smart trousers, or a skirt of decent length, and a smart top of some description, or a suit and shirt, will be regarded as suitable. If you don't have such things in your wardrobe then it's worth getting them – it is a small cost in comparison to 5 or 6 years at medical school, and you will need them again anyway. You should avoid jeans, way out clothing, too much in the way of facial and ear piercing, and overpowering aftershaves and perfumes. Imagine what you would like your doctor to look like when you go and see him/her. This is not to say that you must not wear more casual clothes but why take unnecessary chances?

Before the interview

You will often be waiting around for several hours and sometimes more than 1 day to be interviewed. There will be lots of other candidates who are all as nervous as you. Try to remain calm. There is usually lots of talk about other interviews, what A levels you are doing/have done, whether you have offers from other universities, and lots of tall stories about the questions that people got asked in previous years/interviews. It is easy to let this worry you but try not to get rattled.

When it is time for your interview, make sure that you are early. If you arrive late, you will be flustered and unable to present yourself in the best way, and it creates a bad impression. Get to the place where the interviews are being held in good time and wait quietly outside. This will allow you time to prepare yourself.

Preparation on the day of the interview

- Dress and look like a doctor
- Know where you need to be and when
- Be early
- Remain calm
- Don't let others panic you

What do the interviewers know about you before the interview?
All the interviewers will have received photocopies of your UCAS form. On this are your personal details such as name, age and address; your qualifications, and the subjects that you are planning to take; your personal statement; and a reference from your head teacher/teachers/sponsor. Often the reference is written by your teachers and then the head teacher will write an introduction and conclusion. Usually teachers write what grade you are predicted to get in each subject. The medical school will take any negative comments seriously. The interviewers will not be aware of your other UCAS choices because these are removed before the form is sent to the University.

7.4 The interview itself

The structure of the interview(s)
Usually you will have one or two interviews and there will be two or three people in the interview panel, although sometimes there may be more. The interviewers will be a mix of academics (who teach basic sciences in the undergraduate curriculum) and clinicians (such as GPs and hospital doctors). In addition there may be a medical student on the panel. The interviews are usually about 20–30 minutes long.

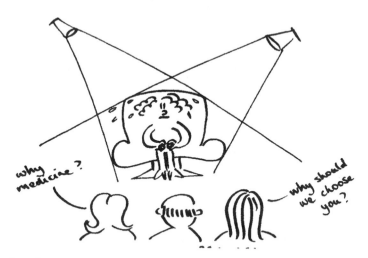

The interview process

Interview etiquette
By this we mean how you should present yourself during the interview. Remember that body language contributes about 70% of communication,

that is to say, 70% of communication is non-verbal. How you look and behave can be as important as what you say!

On arrival you will be introduced to the panel of interviewers. Shake hands with the panel if you are given the chance, look them in the eye and say, 'Good morning' or 'Good afternoon' or 'Hello' as appropriate. Wait to be invited to sit down in the correct chair.

When sitting, adopt an interested posture – sitting upright in the chair, leaning forward slightly and looking ready for the first question. Do not loll in the chair as if you are watching TV at home. Do not cross your legs. Do not fidget or fiddle with things in your pockets or hands – even if you are nervous. These things are all distracting and irritating for the interviewers. Make sure that you speak clearly and at a reasonable pace – don't babble or waffle! Listen carefully to the question and answer the question you are asked, not the one you would rather answer! At the end of the interview you should stand up and shake hands before leaving.

What are they looking for?

Interviewers are looking for students who are academically capable, well motivated and show the appropriate attributes of a doctor.

The following tables are examples of attributes that interviewers are trying to assess. This format is used at Oxbridge, where a candidate would have two interviews, but aspects from these tables will be used to assess students at all interviews.

Academic potential interview

Candidate's name:

Criterion	Score (where a = first rate; b = good; c = average; d = below average; e = very weak)
Reasoning ability: ability to analyse and solve problems using logical and critical approaches	
Originality and creativity of thought: lateral thinking and hypothesis generation	
Speed of thinking and responding	
Spirit of enquiry: keenness to understand the reason for observations; depth; tendency to look for meaning; enthusiasm and curiosity in science	
Observation: accurate, critical, quantitative	

(Continued)

Academic potential interview (*Continued.*)

Candidate's name:

Criterion	Score (where a = first rate; b = good; c = average; d = below average; e = very weak)
Communication: in a tutorial context; willingness and ability to express clearly and effectively; ability to listen; compatibility with tutorial format	
Other factors	
Overall assessment: (taking above into account but not following a strict algorithm)	

Medicine suitability interview

Candidate's name:

Criterion	Score (where a = acceptable; u = unacceptable)
Empathy: ability and willingness to imagine the feelings of others and understand the reasons for the views of others	
Motivation: a reasonably well informed and strong desire to practise medicine	
Communication: ability to clarify knowledge and ideas using language appropriate to the audience	
Honesty and integrity	
Ethical awareness	
Other factors: ability to work with others; capacity for sustained and intense work	
Overall assessment	

7.5 What are you going to be asked?

This is the big question! Every year the interviewers try to think of new questions that they can ask the candidates to try and test them. In general they will start by trying to put you at ease. It is usual for one of the interviewers to run through aspects of your personal statement. This is why it is important to study a copy before interview and also why it is essential not to lie or exaggerate.

Following this they will move on to more general questioning, which could be divided into various topics as set out below. Of course it is impossible to guarantee that these are the questions that you will be asked, but these suggestions have been included to stimulate further thought.

Medical questions

About your choice of medicine and medical school:
- Why do you want to be a doctor?
- Did anyone you know influence your choice of career?
- Do you have family members who are doctors? What do they think of the field? How have their lives changed over the past few years with the changes in medicine? Do you want to follow in their footsteps?
- Which field of medicine are you interested in?
- Why did you apply to our university?
- Are you aware of the differences in our course, compared to other courses? Do you think these should be changed? How would you change them?
- Why should we choose you?
- What are your strengths and weaknesses? What would you change about yourself?
- What qualities would you look for in a doctor?

About the NHS:
- What are the principles of the NHS?
- Do you think that the NHS will exist when you qualify?
- How would you fund healthcare in this country?
- What do you think is the most difficult issue facing the medical community?
- Do you think those who can afford private medical cover should be forced to have it?
- Tell me about a recent media issue involving the NHS.
- Do you know of any changes in the future training of doctors?
- If you can afford it, do you think you should be able to get better care by going privately?

Ethical issues:
- If you find that the professor with whom you have done research has changed some of the data before publication, what would you do?
- What would you do if you saw a fellow medical student/friend cheating in an exam?
- If an HIV positive patient was bleeding profusely from a laceration, what would you do? What if you do not have gloves? What if you have an open sore on your hands?

- Should smokers be offered the same rights to treatment as non-smokers? What if they refuse to give up?
- What do you understand by euthanasia? Does euthanasia have a role in modern medicine?
- What do you think of herbal/alternative medicine? Should people choose them over traditional medicine? What would you do if a family member decides to depend solely on alternative medicine for his treatment of a significant illness (cancer, etc.)?
- Convince me that smoking cannabis should be made legal.

Science questions:
These are infinite in their scope. Some examples are listed below:
- If I release a balloon full of air and allow it to go flying around the room, draw a graph of pressure in the balloon against time.
- What is 12 times 16? How did you calculate this?
- Why do we have seasons?
- Why is it harder to breath at altitude?
- How do bicycle gears work?
- Do mitochondria have DNA? Why/why not? Could they reproduce in isolation?
- Discuss something that you know a lot about.

The interviewers are not looking to see if you have previously learnt the answers to these questions, they are trying to see if you can work out the answer by logical thought, they will usually guide you through if necessary. They want to see how you approach the questions.

Sometimes props will be used, for example, a bone, a surgical instrument or an X-ray. Again you are not expected to know everything but to be able to talk in a sensible and constructive way.

Extracurricular activities:
- Do you plan to continue your hobbies through medical school?
- If you had 1 day to do anything, what would you do?
- What was the last book you read? What did you think about it? Would you recommend that I read it? The last movie you saw? What did you think of it?
- Who do you admire the most in your life? If you could chose one figure in history to have dinner with, who would it be?

Any questions?
Finally, you are likely to be asked whether you have any questions for the interviewers. You do not have to have any. It is perfectly acceptable to say,

'No, thank you, I have been on the open day and spoken with other students and all my questions have been answered' or something similar. It is better not to ask a question that you should have found the answer to at the open day. If you do have a sensible question, you should ask it, but don't ask something pathetic just for the sake of asking a question.

7.6 Differences at Oxford and Cambridge

First of all you can apply to either Cambridge or Oxford only – not both! See Chapter 6 for further details.

Oxford exam

In the past there was an Oxford entrance exam which was sat in schools. This was abolished about 10 years ago and for several years candidates sat an exam in Oxford when they attended for interview. This changed again in 2003. All applicants to Oxford (along with several other medical schools) now sit the BMAT (BioMedical Admissions Test) exam (see Chapter 3). Following successful interview candidates are now given a conditional offer like everywhere else.

Cambridge

Cambridge did not have an entrance exam for many years and relied on interviews and conditional offers. A few years ago it started to use the MVAT (Medical and Veterinary Admissions Test) but this was replaced in 2003 by the BMAT.

The Interviews

Traditionally the interviews at Oxford and Cambridge have been much more academic than other institutions. Either one or both of the interviews may be dedicated to testing the candidates' academic skills and lateral thinking. The questions are not supposed to see how much you know but instead how much you can work out for yourself (see the Science questions section, pp 72). Often the topics are based on things that you should know about, but then try to push you to the next step. Candidates find this worrying and can be easily thrown off their guard. The nature of these questions means that you cannot prepare for them easily. Remember that everyone is in the same position. Try to remain calm, don't panic and think through your answer. The interviewers are trying to assess how you think! Take your time in answering and don't blurt out the first thing that comes into your head!

When you apply to Oxford or Cambridge you may specify to which colleges you wish to apply or make an open application (the University will allocate you to a college). Provided you meet the academic requirements of the college and pass the BMAT exam, it is likely that you will be interviewed. You will probably have two interviews at any given college. Most colleges now have a 'medical suitability' interview as well as a traditional academic interview at Oxbridge.

Remember that not all colleges have the same number of applicants. The more popular/famous colleges tend to have greater numbers of applicants and this increases the competition. You can find out how many applicants each college received for each subject from the university and college prospectuses.

7.7 The future

Traditionally, selection of medical students has been based almost entirely on academic success. Owing to the number of excellent applicants outweighing the number of places, this has led over the years to the gradual increase in the A level standards required in order to gain a place at medical school. Even over the last 10 years the average offer has risen from BBB to AAB. This situation may lead to some candidates applying for medicine because of their academic ability rather than their actual motivation for the subject. The admissions tests have been introduced in recent years to try and discriminate between candidates and assess their suitability for medicine. However, the interview process will probably remain an assessment of academic potential and personality in most universities.

7.8 Finally

Statistically, you have a reasonably good chance of getting into medical school (approx. 2.5 applications per place in 2005). Also there are more opportunities to enter medical school at later dates either as a mature student or as a graduate student on a 4 year course. There are more medical schools and many more medical students now than ever before due to the opening of new medical schools and the increases in the number of medical school places at the other universities. Medicine is a rewarding and fulfilling career, but is also very tough and requires long hours of learning, numerous exams and hard work. Think carefully, do your homework and apply!

Chapter 8 **Over 21s**

We have entitled this chapter Over 21s, as the terminology for the older student applying for medicine can become confusing. The first thing to do is to distinguish between mature students and graduate students. Mature students are those who are older than the usual school leavers (over 21), but who haven't studied for a previous degree. Graduate students are those who have studied for a previous degree and then decide to study medicine. Both groups may be subdivided into those that have done science A levels (or equivalent) or a science degree, and those that have not. There is officially no maximum age for applying to medical school, but as a rule the universities have to take into account how many years after qualifying you will be able to offer as a doctor, and you must be realistic about the cost of training and the potential limits in your career progression if you start at an older age. This chapter should be used in combination with the course code tables at the end of Chapter 2 and the table at the end of Chapter 5 showing entry requirements and additional courses on offer for graduate students and mature students without a science background (Figure 8.1).

8.1 Applications

Applications are through UCAS – using the same form as school leavers. You can enter 4 choices of medical school, and it is important that you choose courses for which you are eligible. If you are a graduate you may enter some 4-year and some 5-year course choices. You will also need a reference from your current employer, or if you are a graduate, from a recent tutor. You must indicate in your personal statement why you want to apply for medicine, why you didn't apply previously and why you think you would be suited to the course. If you applied as a school leaver and were not accepted at that time then you should indicate what has changed since then.

You will need to demonstrate that you have investigated your choice thoroughly. If you are not currently working in a healthcare field then you must demonstrate that you have been interested and involved in medicine. The

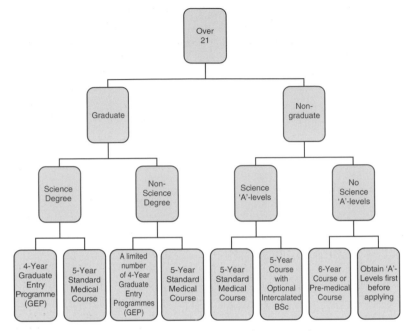

Figure 8.1 Medical degree options for graduate and mature students.

most common method is through voluntary work. There are a huge number of organisations that would be grateful for your time and will provide you with experience. Examples include hospice voluntary work, hospital volunteering, St John's ambulance, Samaritans, working as a nurse auxiliary/healthcare assistant, working on social/welfare committees either at university or as community work, working with physically or mentally disabled people, volunteering at a nursing home, shadowing hospital staff or GPs, and working for charities overseas.

8.2 Graduate students

In 2005, 21% of all first year medical students in England were graduates studying medicine as a second degree. Graduate students who wish to apply for medicine must have achieved at least a 2:1 in their first degree to be seriously considered to study at medical school. Graduates can choose to enter a 'standard' 5-(or 6) year medical degree but it is now more attractive to try and enter a 4-year graduate entry programme (GEP). Four-year GEPs have been available since 2000 and have been expanded to include many medical schools. Most still require a science degree for entry but many are now including non-science graduates. There are several advantages to a GEP over a standard course. Firstly, and most obviously, the course is shorter and therefore you will start earning sooner. Secondly, the Department of Health will pay the tuition fees for the 2nd–4th years of the 4-year graduate entry courses, whereas it will only pay for the 5th (and 6th) years of a standard course for graduate entrants. Also graduates are not eligible for loans for tuition fees and because the tuition fees will be £3000 per annum this alone is a difference of at least £9000 between the two types of course. Thirdly, there are differences in the student loans available for maintenance: the GEP entrants can claim a full student loan in the first year and then reduced rates in the subsequent 3 years; whereas graduates on a standard course can claim full loans for maintenance in the first 4 years and reduced rates in the 5th (and 6th) years. Finally, GEP entrants can claim Department of Health bursaries in the 2nd–4th years whereas the graduates on the standard courses can only claim them in the 5th (and 6th) years.

Unlike school leavers graduates may apply to both Oxford and Cambridge GEPs. However, the course fees are higher at Oxford and Cambridge (around £4500 per annum in 2006 in Oxford) as they include college as well as university fees.

Apart from being a shorter course the courses are more self-directed, problem-based and have clinical involvement much earlier. It is argued that graduate students are better motivated, but students starting these courses will nonetheless be expected to be very self-motivated and self-disciplined to achieve the same standards in training. These courses are extremely popular with often between 30 and 70 applications per place.

Medical School offering GEP	Approximate number of places	Entrance exam	Degree requirement
Barts and The London Queen Mary's School	40	MSAT	At least 2:1 in a science or health related degree
Birmingham	40	None at present	At least 2:1 in a life science + good knowledge of chemistry (A-level standard)
Bristol	19	None at present	At least 2:1 in a science or health related degree

(Continued)

(*Continued.*)

Medical School offering GEP	Approximate number of places	Entrance exam	Degree requirement
Cambridge	20	BMAT	At least 2:1 in any degree + A-levels in science subjects
Guy's, King's and St Thomas', London	24	MSAT	At least 2:1 in any degree (or 2:2 if also have higher degree)
Leicester	64	UKCAT	At least 2:1 in a science or health related degree
Liverpool	32	None at present	At least 2:1 for Biomedical/Health Science graduates + BBB at A level (incl. Biology and Chemistry)
Newcastle	25	UKCAT	At least 2:1 in a science or health related degree
Nottingham	91	GAMSAT	At least 2:2 in any Honours degree
Oxford	30	UKCAT	At least 2:1 in an experimental science degree
St George's, London	84	GAMSAT	At least 2:2 in any Honours degree
Southampton	40	None at present	At least 2.1 in any degree + a pass at A level in chemistry or passes in biology/human biology and chemistry at AS level or equivalent
Swansea	70	GAMSAT	At least 2:1 in any degree
Warwick	164	MSAT	At least 2:1 in a biological science degree

BMAT: BioMedical Admissions Test; GAMSAT: Graduate Medical School Admissions Test; MSAT: Medical Schools Admissions Test; UKCAT: UK Clinical Aptitude Test.

8.3 Mature students

Mature students are generally treated no differently from school leavers when it comes to getting a place at a university and most universities accept a relatively small number of non-graduate mature students each year. You must fulfil the same entry requirements as the school leavers. If you have a science background, then you must achieve the necessary grades for entry into the university you have chosen. If you are from a non-scientific background, you will need to apply for a course with a built-in premedical year or undergo a recognised 1-year premedical training year (foundation courses). There are now many universities offering 6-year courses with a built-in pre-medical year: Bristol, Cardiff, Dundee, Edinburgh, Keele, King's College London, Manchester, Sheffield and Southampton. There are also 1-year stand-alone courses being run, which if completed successfully, allow you to apply to medical school. Such a course is run at the College of West Anglia based in King's Lynn. It is a full time 1-year course that is currently recognised at 21 medical schools. Recently, 90% of its course leavers entered medical school. There is another access course at Manchester College of Arts and Technology (Access to Medicine, Dentistry and Pharmacy) and The Open University also runs some courses that are recognised for entry into some medical schools. You have to do well (high marks or distinction) in these courses to be considered and there is no guarantee that you will obtain a place at medical school.

If you apply to The Peninsula Medical School (Exeter and Plymouth) as a mature student you will be required to sit the GAMSAT exam. Other medical schools will require you to sit the relevant entrance test (UKCAT or BMAT) accordingly (see Chapter 3).

PERSONAL VIEW   *Marcus Hatch*

In July 2003, I was 31 years old, married, living in a beautiful part of Wiltshire, doing a job I absolutely enjoyed and being paid for it. Life was good.

By October 2003, I was unemployed, I'd bought a house in the East Midlands – wherever the hell that was, I'd moved away from friends, family, and familiarity and even dragged my wife with me.

Why? For a place in the first cohort of Nottingham University's new Graduate Entry Medicine (GEM) course.

Working as a Paramedic was a job I loved doing, however I increasingly came to realise that clinically, it was limited. I could try to seek a management role but that wasn't the kind of people contact that I was looking for. I occasionally floated the idea of becoming a doctor but the prospect of trying to achieve those A-levels, at this stage of my life, was not appealing! I then began to hear of the graduate entry scheme, particularly the one based at St George's, London, which accepted degrees of any flavour, even my International Politics and International History degree. Research revealed that Nottingham was also running

(Continued)

(*Continued*)
a similar course and that they would be sharing the application process with St George's, my chances had doubled! Further research, however, showed surging popularity for these courses as well as the requirement to sit the GAMSAT paper. My chances seemed to be shrinking again!

Regardless, I decided to dip my toe into UCAS' muddy waters and apply. The GAMSAT was in London and lasted from 8.30 am to 5 pm. I left with mixed feelings but 2 months later the results arrived and shortly after I was offered an interview.

The interview was highly structured and scores were applied to the answers to allow transparency between the two medical schools. The interview was tough as there was little latitude from the structure and I left frustrated as I felt they knew no more about me than when I arrived. That said, I was ultimately offered a place.

Accepting the offer brought the inevitable worry and doubt with the sheer logistics of moving 150 miles, losing one income and buying a house in an area we knew nothing about, all within a 3-month timescale. My wife was able to negotiate a change from office working to working from home, which allowed us to maintain that source of income. Full use of student loans, professional studies loan and general belt-tightening has enabled us to still be reasonably comfortable and the NHS Bursary from year 2 onwards pays for fees.

Our cohort of 90 people consisted of roughly equal numbers of arts versus science graduates with previous occupations ranging from students to bankers, lawyers, engineers, health professionals, teachers and a cheese monger. This bizarre collection was placed well away from the undergraduate course in Nottingham, by building a new school within the grounds of Derby City General Hospital. The 18-month preclinical, problem based learning (PBL) was done from here. Personally, I found PBL a good way to learn, one that more suited my style than one based on rote learning. That said, it's not for everyone and if you've locked horns with PBL before and not liked it, think carefully about such a PBL-heavy course as this.

Here we stayed, safe within the 'Derby Old Peoples Home' (those cheeky undergrads!) until halfway through year 2.

At this point, the GEM and the 5-year course come together to share a common clinical training until graduation. This was a time of some trepidation, for us, for the undergrads and for the staff. As it was, I believe it was a smooth transition. There was little hostility and fears that one group or the other would excel in certain areas of knowledge or expertise had little foundation. Writing a year later, I see little difference in knowledge or performance between the two groups,

(*Continued*)

(Continued.)

which is as it should be, as neither course is better or worse at teaching – just different in its approach.

Outside the hospital/classroom, the differences are perhaps more marked. There is less tendency for GEMs to revel in spending a Friday evening drinking flavoured meths from a bucket (known euphemistically as a 'cocktail', presumably more Molotov than margarita), although this is not universally true!

As a GEM student, you have had the hedonistic pleasures of studentdom already, and there is perhaps less excitement in uni life than there was then. Many have family, children and a network of social interests that obviously continue despite being a student again. That said, as the GEMs are themselves so varied, there are exceptions to every rule.

Personally, I have found graduate entry medicine an amazing experience. The course is challenging and long, even if it's 'only' 4 years, and there are definitely times I've thought, 'What am I doing?' Despite this, the promise of a career that will be ever evolving, consistently challenging and regularly rewarding and can follow paths as mainstream or as obscure as you wish, must be seized with both hands.

Chapter 9 **Life at medical school**

9.1 The beginning

There are those who say that school years are the best years of your life. It is likely that these people have never been to university. University, although hard work, can be a great deal of fun. Whatever course you decide to study, there will be many lasting memories. Choosing medicine gives you a longer course, more students, more societies and more social events. The downside is the excess of exams and the longer course meaning increased poverty. A further unique feature is the virtual guarantee of a job following graduation, although with the increase in university places and the recent reduction in training posts this may not be the case in the future (see Chapter 17 for more information).

For many, commencing university will be the first time away from home. Most universities now reserve a place in a hall of residence (or college) for first year students. This is perfect for getting to know other students, both medical and non-medical. No matter what kind of person you are, you will meet

What did I think I knew before I went to university?

- University would be good.
- Medical school would be extremely hard work.
- After 5 years I would qualify and know everything about medicine.
- Working long hours was only for the first year after graduation.
- Exams take place only during university years.
- Medicine is a respected profession.
- Dissection would be disgusting.

What didn't I know before I went to university?

- GP or surgeon – are there other career options available?
- Doctors on call – what does that mean?

people in the first few weeks who will end up being friends for life. Most people will be in the same situation in that they will not know other students before starting. This means that there will be no preconceived opinions regarding your personality before you begin. The advice is just be yourself. The old adage 'children can be so cruel' can be true during school life but once at university the added maturity of students tends to mean teasing and stereotyping are much less common.

9.2 Accommodation

College rooms

As already mentioned, most first year students are reserved a place in a hall of residence. For students applying to Oxbridge this will mean accommodation within the chosen college, and for other universities it will usually mean accommodation fairly close to a central campus and medical school. For those students who are not able to gain a place, do not fear, as most will be found places in alternative accommodation that will have liaisons with the other halls. In advance it is difficult to know what personal belongings to bring with you for that very first day. The rooms may be limited in both size and storage area. Most students are dropped off by their parents on the first day with only essential items and then have several trips back home over the next few weeks to pick up the rest of their stuff. This of course means that at the end of the year you have too much stuff for one carload – it is amazing how much hoarding can occur in only one term!

So you've arrived at what is to be home for the next 10 weeks or so. Once the boxes have been transferred to your new room, it is time to gently encourage the parents and loved ones to wander back. Of course there may be tears, but it is time to discover your new environment and meet new friends. Halls and colleges tend to be arranged in blocks with most students having a single room with shared bathroom facilities and a kitchen. The facilities available in the kitchen will depend on whether your particular residence is catered or whether you will be experiencing such literary classics as 'cooking for students'. The days of single-sex residences are numbered and, as the demand for mixed-sex halls grows, more of the traditional places will no doubt convert. Most halls have central communal areas including a canteen and junior common room (JCR). The JCR is usually the focus for hall life and will have a television and other entertainment such as a pool table and video games. The advantage of living in the university accommodation in your first year is that it is good for getting to meet new friends. It is also reasonably cheap as all bills and quite often food is included. The disadvantages are the size of the accommodation, the lack of privacy and sometimes the quality of the hall canteen.

Renting or buying

Following the first year the majority of students venture away from the security of halls and colleges. During the second and subsequent years it is quite common to live in student houses with between three and six friends. The quality of this accommodation can vary considerably and so can the cost. It is definitely worth viewing several places before making a choice. Bigger groups of students will find limited availability. Many houses in student areas are substandard despite the introduction of rules and regulations regarding quality and safety. The university will set standards and have a database of houses and landlords who comply. The reality is that the demand far outweighs the supply. Some towns now have student developments off campus in blocks of flats, often renovated from old warehouses. These are often in good condition and offer a similar social experience to living in halls in the first year. One option would be to move each year and experience different types of accommodation with various friends.

As medicine is a 5-year course, another option in year 2 would be to buy a property. This could be done with a group of friends or on your own with friends renting from you. This has considerable initial set up costs but could save money in the long run if the value of the house rises. A deposit of at least 10% of the purchase price is usually required and it may be necessary to obtain a loan from your parents or loved ones. The other initial costs include stamp duty, search fees and solicitor fees. As you will not have an income, it will be necessary for a relative to act as a guarantor for your mortgage. The debate about the sort of mortgage to go for (repayment, interest only, ISA etc.) is ongoing, but advice from several financially astute individuals is recommended.

Once out of university accommodation, the cost of living will undoubtedly increase and this has to be remembered when budgeting. Not only will there be rent but also fuel, phone and food bills.

If you decide to rent then once a suitable house is found it is necessary to complete a contract with the landlord. This should be an assured shorthold tenancy agreement. This means that you will be renting the house as a group and so, if one person moves out, the rest of the tenants could be liable to pay their share. The household bills will need to be changed into your own names and you will have the responsibility for payment. Some students buy individual provisions but an alternative option might be to have communal cooking and hence shared food costs. This can work out cheaper as the necessity for a pint of milk for each individual student will be avoided. It can also avoid the inevitable arguments when someone's last egg mysteriously disappears.

As far as choosing your housemates, it should become obvious during the first term who have become your good mates. Of course there can still be teething problems and some students do swap houses in the following years.

The major gripe will be if one or two friends are not pulling their weight with the household chores. In this instance it may be worth creating rotas for cleaning.

Not all students move away from halls or colleges in the second year, and some actually move back in during their final years. Living in hall is certainly the cheaper of the two options but renting in student houses is another experience not to be missed during your university life.

What did I discover during university?

- University was good fun.
- Medical school was not as hard as I imagined.
- After 5 years I would qualify and know everything about medicine – this is just the beginning.
- Working long hours exists for most of your career.
- There are many, many career choices.
- For most careers, postgraduate exams are necessary.
- Medicine is a respected profession.
- On call can be lonely, tiring and scary.
- It is sensible to avoid hangovers on dissection mornings.

Rental survival

There are many horror stories told about naïve students being ripped off by dodgy landlords. In general the majority of students get through their university rental days unscathed. Each university will have a list of approved properties and landlords, and this is a good starting point. This doesn't actually mean that the houses will be luxurious, but means that they must meet certain minimum criteria.

The job of finding a suitable place often requires hours spent tramping the streets, knocking on doors. A slightly quicker method will be to use an agency who can find suitable property for you (they may charge for this service though). Once a house has been found, discuss with the current tenants about what the landlord has been like over the preceding year regarding repairs, popping round uninvited, supplying smoke detectors, etc. If they have been satisfied, then arrange to meet with the landlord. All those intending to move into the property should be present. At this meeting discuss deposit, rent, bills and safety checks, and read a copy of the proposed contract. It is probably worth taking the contract away and reading it carefully before signing. If in any doubt regarding the contents, ask a parent or solicitor. Check with the landlord what the deposit covers and that s/he has the correct safety certificates – at minimum there should be a gas safety certificate. Houses should also be fitted with fire doors, mains smoke alarms and fire retardant furniture (check the labels) – again this can be uncommon. On the signing of the contract, it is usual to pay either a deposit or retainer payment. There should be an improvement in the standards of the properties since the introduction of the housing act (April 2006). If your house has 5 or more occupants and 3 or more storeys the landlord must be registered with the local council and pay for a license. There have also been health and safety systems introduced and if you or your parents are in any doubt about the safety of your accommodation (including university halls), then you can contact the local housing authority if there is no solution to the problem following discussion with the landlord.

When you move into your new home it is essential to check through the inventory that the landlord should have issued. Make sure you agree before signing. If there is any obvious damage, then note it down – a useful tip is to take some digital photos that can be reviewed at the end of the year. All the bills need to be converted into your own name, although in some circumstances – for example water services – the landlord may be responsible. Students are exempt from council tax.

At the end of the year, inform the landlord of your date of leaving and clean and tidy the house. Your landlord should then come and inspect the property. Following this you should be refunded a proportion of your deposit. The amount of money lost will depend on the condition of the house. If you feel that the landlord has been unfair, then it is time to study the inventory and dig out the digital photos with the evidence (make sure they are dated at the time and countersigned by a friend if necessary). If the landlord does not return the money, then it may be necessary to write to ask for reasons, then possibly seek legal help. From October 2006 a new scheme to protect deposits is being introduced. Landlords will need to take out a special insurance or hand the deposit to a third party. In this way any disputes should be able to be resolved more easily. Any further advice is outside the remit of this chapter and more detailed information can be found at http://www.nusonline.co.uk.

Rental survival tips

- Check the university recommended properties.
- Check the landlord has a license (if applicable).
- Discuss any issues with the current tenants.
- Check the contract carefully before signing.
- Check safety issues (furniture, alarms, gas checks, etc.).
- Request receipts for all payments made.
- Check inventory carefully, take photos, and get witnesses.
- Check the landlord is insured *but* get your own personal room insurance.

9.3 Freshers' week

The emphasis during the first few weeks at university is not really on working at the books but working on the social life. You will only ever experience one freshers' week, so make the most of it. The week consists of settling in and wandering around getting to know your new university and city. Freshers' fayre takes place during the first few days and is usually found in one of the central campus buildings where the students' union has its home. This involves stalls of all the university clubs and societies that you can wander around at your leisure. There tends to be a diverse number of clubs and examples are included in the following table. Representatives from other companies such as banks, pubs, restaurants and nightclubs also attend these first few days. It is possible to pick up a few freebies at this event but be wary of taking your cheque book on the first day because it involves cash to join most of the societies. It is a great chance to try out a new sport, for example, water skiing, but it is unlikely that you will have the time to try out four new sports during your first year. Our advice would be to wander round on the first day and keep your money safely tucked away. Have a look at what is on offer and decide how to spend your money ready for the next visit.

During this first week the university will hold events on most of the nights. These will usually revolve around the university bars and then some of the pubs and clubs in town. All the events held are usually cheap and cheerful with the main aim of getting to know new friends. From the social side of things this week often culminates in a university-wide social event, which could have famous live bands headlining and many other types of entertainment.

9.4 The students' union

The NUS (National Union of Students) was set up in 1922. Today the NUS continues to campaign for student rights and offers support to over 700 students' unions across the country. Each university will have its own students' union. These are the backbone of the NUS and are integral to student life. They provide a broad range of services from welfare advice and information to clubs and societies, bars, shops and catering services, and charity fundraising events. Students' unions also play a vital role in facilitating the representation of students' views within the university. Students' union officers often sit on the board of governors of the college or university and help student course representatives at a departmental level as well as supporting students in academic appeals.

Elected student officers conduct the affairs of the students' union and implement policy. Every student has the opportunity to take part in making decisions on policy and areas of work through general meetings or elected councils. In larger students' unions, some elected officers spend a sabbatical

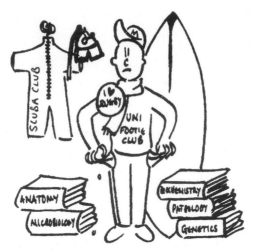

Try and avoid wasting money on too many textbooks or university societies in the first few weeks

Examples of university clubs and societies

- Afro-Caribbean Society
- Anglican Society
- Bike Club
- Bridge Society
- Canoe Society
- Cocktail Society
- Dance Society
- Darts Club
- Folk Dancing
- Food Society
- Golf Society

- Hiking Club
- Lesbian, Gay & Bisexual Society
- Medieval Society
- Movie Society
- Rock Society
- Skiing Society
- Surfing Society
- Swimming Club
- Water Skiing Club
- Windsurfing Society

year working full time for the students' union whilst many unions also employ professional staff. Students' unions decide whether they wish to affiliate to the NUS. Every constituent member of NUS pays an annual subscription fee, which can vary depending on the number of full-time and part-time students who are members of the union, and the amount of money the union receives from their college or university. The funds raised from affiliation fees are used to fund the campaigns and activities of the NUS.

The students' union building for each university will normally be found in a central location. The students' union card can be obtained at various allocated places during the first few weeks. You obviously have to provide proof that you are in full-time education. In return for a small fee the card gives you discounts in various shops, pubs, clubs, restaurants and other organisations, for example rail and air travel.

9.5 The medical school facilities

Universities have strict guidelines to follow, to enable them to set up a medical school. For that reason their actual facilities should not really bother potential applicants too much. Instead of looking round each of the laboratories, time would be more profitably spent chatting to current students, doctors and academics, or even looking around the rest of the university campus and town.

Medical school facilities

- *Faculty office:* Each of the courses at university will be affiliated to a faculty. The faculty office is open during office hours and has many different purposes and personnel. They distribute timetables, organise the exams and generally sort out most problems (or point in the right direction!) that students come across.
- *Histology labs*: Usually kitted out with microscopes for studying science at a cellular level.
- *Clinical skills labs*: A new initiative for many universities. These facilities allow practical skills to be carried out in a controlled environment, using models (for example, taking blood from a model arm). Many of the skills that medical students previously acquired by direct patient contact on the ward will now be practised in such environments.
- *Library*
- *Computing facilities*
- *Dissection room*
- *Physiology labs*
- *Biochemistry labs*
- *Cafeteria*
- *Bookshop*
- *Lecture theatres*
- *Seminar rooms*
- *Common room*

9.6 The first lecture

Of course we shouldn't get too carried away with only socialising in the first week because it is also necessary to begin the medical course. While many of your compatriots may not start lectures in the first week, as a medical student you will not be afforded this luxury. By the first day of lectures you will probably have already met several other medical students and you will now meet up to make your way to the medical school where you will spend most of the next 2 years. The first day will be spent signing on for the course and being shown around the place. Most medical schools have a system in place where you are allocated a 'mum' or 'dad' from the year above. You will normally meet these people on that first day and this may well involve a trip to the local medics' pub. They can advise on all sorts of aspects of medical school. Some will sell you their old textbooks and give you various hints and tips along the way regarding exams and course work. Of course they also know the good pubs, restaurants and where to hang around in your new city.

Before you arrive at university it is possible that you will have been sent a starter pack filled with useful information and suggestions for possible purchases. It is easy to get carried away with buying lots of textbooks either before you begin the course or in the first few weeks. Some people even buy equipment such as ophthalmoscopes. This is not to be encouraged and will work out to be very costly. Most of the books will end up collecting dust on your shelves and become out of date quickly. There is a considerable market for second hand books which can be a cheap way of obtaining relevant texts, but a word of caution: ask yourself why the second year student is selling before buying out of date and unhelpful texts. Alternatively the library is a very useful resource and will have multiple copies of the most popular books. In my experience I bought lots of books in the first year, which I regretted, and indeed they did collect dust. Following this I chose more carefully and used the library and also swapped books with friends who were doing different attachments at different times. The advice regarding equipment such as a stethoscope will depend on whether the university you are joining runs a clinical course or a more traditional-based lecture course for the first 2 years. Anything more advanced than a stethoscope will not be necessary. Everything you need you will be able to buy in the first few days once you have arrived at university.

9.7 The medical society

We have already mentioned the various university clubs. As a medical student you are eligible to join the university medical society. This is run by medical students and is exclusively for medical students. The majority of medical students join this society and although membership is not compulsory, it is good value for money. The medical society will have other clubs under its wings, meaning that in your first year it is possible to play sport for your hall of residence/college, medical society or, if you are good enough, the university itself. The medical society also holds regular events that will be subsidised. These will

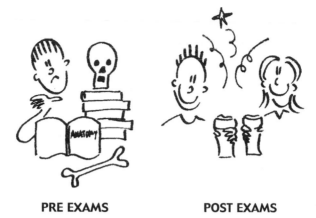

PRE EXAMS   POST EXAMS

Life at medical school

include social events as well as second hand book sales and elective evenings. Second or third year students will normally sit on the committees who are in charge of the clubs and societies that you decide to join. Obviously many of them need enthusiastic first year students to get involved with the organisation at an early stage and possibly continue with more responsible roles later.

9.8 Charity events

During the autumn it is traditional for most universities to take part in raising money for charity. This period of time is known as rag week and consists of rag raids and further social events for raising money. Rag raids involve visiting nearby cities and collecting money by the sale of rag mags (similar to comics). There is the opportunity to join the charity committees or just do your bit by attending the events.

9.9 The social side

Despite the full working week for medics and the amount of study necessary to pass the exams, most students manage to find spare time to enjoy themselves. How this is filled will depend on the individual. Music and sport are two major pastimes that most students will take part in, to some degree. For the adventurous, this may involve starting a new hobby from the many on offer at the freshers' fayre (see earlier examples). Others may continue their current interests and for some it may even be possible to take these to a higher standard, possibly representing the university or even their country – several athletes in the recent Olympic and Commonwealth Games were current medical students or doctors. Having said this, to pursue an activity to such a high standard will require support and understanding from your university or work place. It is sometimes possible to extend your studies or arrange flexible training jobs. Some students may find that they do not have enough time to commit to such a high standard and so continue their interests but more as a way of relaxing.

Sport and music aside, there are many other activities to try while at university and more information can be gained at the freshers' fayre. It has to be said that most of the social events will involve alcohol. For most there will be many drunken tales to tell once university has finished – most of them no doubt embarrassing. Do take care as there can be a fine line between harmless fun and people getting hurt. The other point to remember is that, although it is reasonably difficult to fail medical school, it is still possible, and it would be a shame for a talented medical student to be asked to leave because they didn't know when the partying should have stopped.

9.10 In times of trouble

Of course, for some, the advent of moving away from loved ones does not carry the expected excitement. Some students do find themselves unhappy and this can become even more problematic with a potentially stressful course such as medicine. It is important not to bottle your feelings up. Initially, it will be worthwhile discussing problems with any close friends. If the problems are too personal for this, then a student should approach their nominated course tutor. Not all students get on with their tutor, but most will have found an academic or clinician in whom they can confide. It is possible that the situation may be more serious and, in this case, visiting your GP would be recommended (make sure you register with a new surgery near the university). For those after a confidential ear, most universities provide a telephone service, manned by volunteers. This service often runs in the evenings. Through these channels it is possible to arrange counselling services. Remember that whatever the problem, it is unlikely that it is unique and there will be many people around to discuss the issues – just don't leave it too late.

9.11 Summary

Although often forgotten by more senior doctors, careers advisors and those speaking at courses – UNIVERSITY IS GREAT FUN. The odds are that you will have a good time at whichever university you choose but there is no doubt that medicine can be hard work with lots of exams and assessments.

Medical students do, however, have a bit of a reputation (well deserved), for knowing how to have a good time. Despite the hard work, it is certainly possible to pursue other pastimes and sports. The old saying 'work hard, play hard' is certainly true. One important piece of advice is that it is essential to have interests outside medicine in order to relax.

PERSONAL VIEW   *Rebecca Herbertson*

Like most people who end up at medical school, I had worked pretty hard at school and when I finally got there I was very pleased. I'm not really sure what expectations I had for what would be the next 5 years of my life, but I don't think I could have ever imagined what a great time I would have and what great people I was to meet.

I was soon to get a taste of the medic sense of humour as I was reeled in hook, line, and sinker by those in the year above me on my first day. After finding an official letter under my door on my first night in halls, I was told to produce a urine sample for collection at induction the next morning. Owing to the fact they had apparently run out of urine sample pots I was to bring it in any container that I could find. It took me a long time to admit to anyone that I had actually carried round a camera film container of urine in my bag all day (and surprise, surprise no one really wanted a urine sample at all!).

There is no doubt that it was hard work – not being one of the lucky people who could cruise exams with only a glance at a book, I put the hours in when it came to the all too frequent end of term exams. Seventy-six exams (and a fair few re-takes) later and I was through the first 2 years in medical training. The hours we put in at our desks were certainly equalled by those spent socialising. The third year was a mix of research, organising events as the medical society social secretary and starting life on the wards. White coats, stethoscopes and of course patients made everything much more relevant in the fourth and fifth years. Delivering babies, learning to take blood, holding a retractor in the operating theatre or trying to entertain a child long enough to listen to its chest – I learnt it all during the various attachments, which eventually culminated in qualifying as a doctor!

One of the best aspects of life at medical school was the people I met. Training to become a doctor is a pretty unique experience and the people that you share this with will turn out to be life-long friends. From poring over textbooks together and overdosing on Pepsi-Max, staying up into the small hours revising, unwinding over copious cocktails from plastic dustbins, just about escaping death from an extremely irate hippo in Zimbabwe, to getting decked out in black tie for the graduation ball...my university mates and I have been through it all together, and, without being too cheesy, that's what made it for me!

Chapter 10 **The medical course – early years**

The first edition of this book split the following two chapters into 'the pre-clinical years' and 'the clinical years'. Traditionally the term preclinical referred to the first couple of years at university. During this time the aim is to teach the fundamental knowledge and principles of medicine, in readiness for the later clinical years spent on the wards. The distinction used to be clear, with little of the preclinical time spent out of the lecture theatre, laboratory and dissection room. These terms tend to now be used less with the advent of most medical schools having introduced more modern curricula, with the main aim of students developing clinical skills at an earlier stage, hence the term integrated course. The aim is to familiarise the student with patients, hospital wards and clinical concepts, allowing the students to realise the applicability and relevance of what they are learning in the lecture theatre, through hospital visits and patient contact. Unfortunately, this does not mean you have to learn less! The extent of integration varies between medical schools and it is essential to read the prospectus carefully before applying. There are those who believe that early patient contact is irrelevant as the students have too little knowledge, but we believe this to be a useful exercise, as communicating and dealing with patients and relatives is one of the most essential attributes of a future doctor. Having early patient contact allows essential skills to be learned whilst the student is under careful supervision.

10.1 Mentor/educational supervisor

On arrival at most medical schools, each student is allocated a mentor. This will usually be an academic teacher from one of the affiliated departments (for example, biochemistry). Some students may have the same mentor, who should arrange several meetings over the first couple of years. These get-togethers are to check that you have no particular problems and are progressing with the course, and they often involve feedback following exams. Meetings on a one-to-one basis can be arranged if problems are a little more personal.

10.2 Types of teaching

Regardless of the nature of the course, teaching takes place in the following forms: lectures, practical sessions, dissection, clinical skills sessions and small group tutorials.

Lectures

Formal lectures remain the most common method of teaching. It is usually the easiest way of delivering a large amount of information to large numbers of students. The lectures are usually presented by academics using slides or computer presentations. Handouts may be provided to complement the talks. The format and quality can vary significantly: a university academic does not necessarily have any teaching qualifications. Lectures are becoming less popular as newer methods of teaching are being adopted.

Practical sessions

To help with understanding certain concepts, time will be spent in the laboratory. Here it is possible to apply some of the knowledge gained from the lecture theatre. Practicals undertaken will include subjects such as physiology, biochemistry, pharmacology and microbiology. Occasionally an academic teacher will run the experiment but more often than not it is time for students to get their hands dirty (hopefully not literally, especially for some microbiology experiments!). The particularly fun sessions will involve clinically relevant experiments that can be performed on each other. One of the less pleasant tasks could be inserting a nasogastric tube (tube passed into the stomach) to aid in the measurement of gastric pH. The practical sessions will often involve a write-up following the experiment – in a similar format to those written during A levels. These may count towards a final assessment.

Clinical skills sessions

Most medical schools now have clinical skills laboratories that can be used by students from all years. In these environments it is possible to practice practical skills e.g. taking blood, and also get experience of managing acute medical conditions e.g. cardiopulmonary resuscitation, using mechanical and computerised mannequins and models. With the improvement in technology some of these mannequins are quite advanced – their pupils constrict and dilate, they have palpable pulses and audible breath sounds. These facilities give students the opportunity to improve their skills in a non-threatening environment before carrying them out on real life patients. The clinical sessions will also involve visits to GP surgeries and hospital wards.

Dissection sessions

Ah, the smell of formaldehyde! It's not all lectures during the first couple of years. A major part of the preclinical curriculum is anatomy. The study of anatomy can vary from school to school so it is worth checking on this before arriving. The options include: small group teaching with a donated cadaver which the students dissect, small group teaching using pro-sections (parts of the body previously dissected to show off the relevant parts) or teaching using computer generated images. The best approach will involve a combination. Although we do not recommend purchasing too many textbooks, a good anatomy book and also possibly an anatomy atlas will be necessary. The best approach is to read the relevant chapters before the session and so reinforce the information.

Utmost respect should be paid at all times to the cadavers. These people have kindly donated their bodies for the sake of science. There are many tales that are told to junior medical students regarding the tricks that have been played in the past (placing parts of the bodies in your mate's dinner!). Many are urban myths – if any are true then it is highly inappropriate behaviour. The medical school authorities will take a strict approach with any student caught fooling around and expulsion would be likely.

Another point to remember is that anatomy is relevant and interesting to everybody, not just the budding surgeon.

Tutorials

The problem with lectures is the sheer size of the audience. The disadvantages are that the talks tend to be less interactive and students can feel more intimidated in a crowd and so not ask as many questions. It would be impossible to teach the whole medical school curriculum by tutorials. On arrival at university,

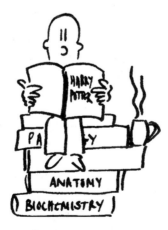

The preclinical years

students will be split into tutorial groups who will meet with a supervisor up to once a week. At these sessions it will be possible to cover problem areas or present experimental findings. It is also likely that, as students, you will be expected to prepare presentations and hand in assignments. It will depend on which medical school as to how much work is involved. The size of tutorials varies greatly between institutions e.g. at Oxford there may only be two students in each group. Schools that run problem-based learning (PBL) courses tend to have more tutorial work.

10.3 Computing

Over the last decade the increase in computer technology has led to the development of increased emphasis being placed on information technology within the medical school curriculum. Universities will now provide teaching on the use of word processing, presentation, statistics, spreadsheet and database packages. Some aspects of the course may be taught using computer-aided learning (CAL) packages to supplement the lecture material. A more recent development is the use of the so-called learning environments where the timetables and objectives for the whole of the medical course are found on Intranet sites. These sites may also provide lecture material, useful links and sample exam questions. Some centres even run certain assessments on the Intranet. Your future career will require increasing use of the Internet and IT methods. While at university take the opportunities available to familiarise yourself with presenting talks using presentation packages and perform literature searches using search engines such as Medline.

10.4 Traditional or modular course

Courses that are more traditional run various subjects each term, for example the first term may consist of a biochemistry module; the second term a physiology module. This trend is changing and the new method is to teach on a whole system, so, for example, in the first term the topic may be the heart. During this first term the physiology, anatomy, biochemistry, and other topics would be taught all relevant to that system. During this time it is common for several hospital visits to be arranged to attempt to put the theoretical knowledge into place with real life patients. The idea is to simplify the course and make everything more relevant.

10.5 The curriculum

Most medical schools introduce the curriculum over the first 2 years in themes. These themes vary between centres but will include in some way, basic medical

sciences, personal and professional development, patient and doctor relationships, public health and community medicine. Basic medical science is the
understanding of the science behind disease processes. Initially it will be necessary to gain an understanding of the normal functioning of the human body
before progressing to the abnormal processes that can occur. This topic is large
and will include biochemistry, physiology, pharmacology, anatomy and microbiology. Unlike school days where the emphasis is around being spoon-fed, at
university you will be expected to cover much of the bookwork in your own
time based around the lectures and tutorials that are presented. The other
themes introduce, at an early part in the course, communication skills, evidence based medicine, population medicine, patient doctor relationships and
psychological aspects related to illness. Universities differ greatly in the amount
of written work that you are expected to complete and hand in for assessment
during the term time. Students at more traditional courses may find more
assessments of this sort during the term. Other medical schools have few or no
essays and practical assignments to be written up, and use the examinations as
the only formal assessment. Again, it is important, when deciding to which
university to apply, that you are aware of the course differences. This can be
achieved by reading the appropriate prospectus and talking to students who
are already studying at the particular institution. You may have to work harder
at some medical schools compared with others!

The early curriculum

- Anatomy
- Biochemistry
- Cytology
- Embryology
- Epidemiology
- Genetics
- Haematology
- Histology

- Immunology
- Microbiology
- Pathology
- Pharmacology and therapeutics
- Physiology
- Psychology
- Sociology

Anatomy

This is the study of body structure and is one of the very essences of medicine, but unfortunately presents a huge amount of information to learn. It is
taught mainly in the lecture theatre and dissection room, but increasingly
through small group tutorials and computer-aided teaching packages. This
subject also involves histology, which is the microscopic appearance of the

different parts of the body, and embryology, which is the study of the development of the human body.

Pathology

Just when you have learnt how everything works and where it is in the body, you have to learn that everything can go wrong, and in many different ways! Pathology is the scientific study of the nature of disease and its causes, processes, development and consequences. It is taught usually through lectures, but also involves attending post mortems and microscope practical sessions.

Pharmacology

Defined as the study of the changes produced in living animals by chemical substances. Often taught with pharmacy students, this course will teach the mechanisms of action of therapeutic agents within the body and their effects, both positive and negative.

Physiology and biochemistry

This is the biological study of the functions of living organisms and their parts and the study of the chemical substances and vital processes occurring in living organisms, respectively. Essentially it is learning about biological processes and how they occur within the human body. The subjects are taught mainly in the lecture theatre, but study also usually involves small group tutorials and practical sessions. Again there is a large amount of information to learn.

10.6 The early clinical experience

It was in the early 1990s with the advent of some newer courses that it was felt earlier clinical exposure was probably useful for medical students. Initially this meant that a handful of schools made a token attempt to integrate the course, which often just meant a brief visit to a hospital ward each term. This has become more formalised over the last decade especially with the opening of the newer establishments. The majority now run fully integrated courses, although the extent of clinical contact in the first 2 years can vary, so it is worth checking before applying. The experience can vary from a few visits each semester to a local hospital or GP, to a dedicated session each week. As many courses are taught in a system based approach (see above section), hospital visits are often organised for the relevant system at the appropriate time. As well as the hospital visits, students will often be attached to a local GP surgery for the whole of the 2 years. During this time some universities assign students various community projects e.g. watching the development of a new born baby, following the progress of an older person after surgery. This early exposure to patients aims to make the basic medical sciences more relevant to everyday practice. It also assists with students developing their communication skills. As there is now this clinical component to the early years, assessment methods have also changed and students will be required to demonstrate, at an early stage, their competence in various clinical situations (see below).

10.7 Problem-based learning (PBL)

When applying to medical school you will have considered the merits of each different university and course. Some applicants may be concerned with the range of bars, others with the ratio of boys to girls. As discussed earlier another decision to bear in mind is the type of course, and a concept that you should all be aware of is self-directed PBL.

At school a common teaching technique is the spoon-feeding method. Students are told what to learn and given fact after fact. This way the emphasis on reading around the subject is neglected and there is a tendency to cram the knowledge, in order to pass the exams. Medical education has undergone sweeping changes over the last few years and new methods and ideas for teaching are being introduced.

PBL is not a new concept. Its origins date back to France in 1920, with a teacher (Célestin Freinet) returning from the First World War unable to speak to his pupils for very long before being too short of breath, due to the injuries he sustained. Owing to this disability he developed methods to get his pupils more involved during the classes. His radical methods, despite the encouraging results, were rejected by all establishments until in 1969, McMaster University in Ontario, Canada, adopted PBL, led by Howard Barrows. The University of Maastricht followed in 1974, and many other centres worldwide have since followed suit. From as far afield as Australia and Bahrain, to right here in the UK, PBL is the new face of how you are likely to be taught at some stage during your medical education. This new method is not being limited to medicine; other subjects to change include law, economics and mathematics.

So what is it?
Basically PBL rests on the principle that crammed information given to you in a didactic fashion, and regurgitated for an exam, is soon forgotten. Alternatively, if a student has to search for the information, it is likely to remain in the memory for a longer period of time. This technique is more suited to the

university style of teaching, as information tends no longer to be spoon-fed and the emphasis is more on individual information gathering.

The way it works in reality is by having small group seminars. A university tutor will get together with a group of students (usually between six and ten), and discuss some trigger material, which may be a letter, a video or a fictitious scenario. From that, together as a group and guided by the tutor, you discuss issues raised and come up with some learning objectives for the week. You then break up and gather the information for yourselves from various resources such as books, the Internet, professionals, and each other. When you return after a week, you solve the problems set by sharing all the information you have found, again guided by the tutor. You will often hear this referred to as the adult learning method, and you will learn about the seven or eight step tutorial process.

It all sounds a little touchy-feely compared with what you are used to, but research and experience has shown that qualifying doctors from this type of course are just as capable as their traditionally taught colleagues. They are better equipped to deal with real clinical situations, better communicators and more able to carry the skills on to life-long learning (vital for all doctors owing to the speed of advances in the medical world).

Whether you like it or not, many universities in the UK (such as Manchester) have, or are in the process of adopting PBL into their courses, either in part, or wholeheartedly for the full 5 years. Be aware of this change and be able to express a sensible opinion on the topic if asked at interview. It would be advisable to discuss this type of course with both tutors and students from the practising universities. This is a particular popular method of teaching the graduate courses.

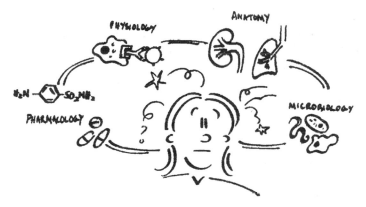

The medical curriculum

10.8 Examinations and assessments

If you have had little experience of exams up until now, then things are about to change. We have mentioned a few of the advantages of being a medical student but by far the biggest disadvantage is the so-called working week and the amount of examinations over the 5 years. When you arrive at university, some of your friends in hall may be enrolled on courses where their working week is only 14 hours. Unfortunately, as a medic, you will have a week consisting of 9–5 every weekday (and at some places possibly even Saturday mornings!). Your friends will, of course, have exams and probably more course work, so it is not all doom and gloom. Starting at medical school may well introduce you to different types of examination formats.

The true/false exam

This is a slight variation on a theme for the multiple choice exam that you will have been familiar with following A levels. It usually involves a stem question followed by several statements. All questions have to be answered and the statement given is either true or false (not exactly rocket science). The problem is that, if you answer incorrectly, then you are deducted a point, the so-called negative marking. There is therefore an option to abstain (don't know). Not all universities use the negative marking system and some may use the multiple choice format rather than true/false. Another similar format is 'best of five' – there is a stem for the question and then you have to pick the answer from 5 options.

The short answer exam and essay exam

This is self-explanatory. It usually requires a bit more studying than the true/false exam.

Viva voce exam

This is an oral exam where you will be questioned on a topic by one or two examiners. These normally last for around 15 minutes. The topics can include physiology and pharmacology. Anatomy is also examined in this way but often will involve the examiners using pro-sections (a dissected part of the body) to focus the discussion.

Practical session

Occasionally some subjects may be examined from a slightly more practical perspective. Examples include histology where various slides will be shown under microscopes; pathology where various frozen sections could be presented, and physiology where you may be required to demonstrate an experiment.

Clinical skills

Traditionally clinical skills were not really assessed during the early part of university. This has changed with the integrated courses and clinical type examination formats are often used even in the first year. These can take the format of OSCE (Objective Structured Clinical Examination) and OSLER (Objective Structured Long Examination Record) assessments. It may be necessary to demonstrate practical skills and patient management but obviously to a lesser ability than would be expected in more senior years. These assessment methods are discussed in detail in Chapter 11.

Other types of assessment

During term time some colleges expect essays to be written following small group tutorials, and practical experiment write-ups to be completed, and this may form part of an assessment, but may not count towards your final exams.

The intercalated degree

This is dealt with in more detail in Chapter 12. It is important to be aware that at some institutions this degree is included as part of the preclinical years, so students will obtain a degree at the end of their third year. Most other universities will allow a certain number of students to defer the start of their clinical years by studying for a degree during a further year following their preclinical. At Cambridge and Oxford, the intercalated degree is compulsory and can be taken in a non-medical speciality.

10.9 Summary

It is not so much the difficulty of the work that some students struggle with at university, but more the sheer volume of information required to learn. It is essential not to get too far behind with your work as it will be difficult to catch up. If you have not done biology at A level, some universities will provide some extra tutorials but in our experience it made no difference to students' success at exams. Whichever course is taught, you will be required to spend a significant amount of time for personal study. Reviewing the university prospectuses is essential as the courses still vary with regard to the amount of PBL and the amount of clinical exposure in the first 2 years. Make the most of the clinical time, as it can be very rewarding. Try not to worry too much about the assessments and just take each step at a time – you no doubt remember thinking A levels would be impossible while you were studying for GCSEs, but you will get through them!

My first memory of Medical School, one hazy September afternoon having said a tearful goodbye to my father, was staring at a crumpled heap of metal wires. The challenge of assembling the newly bought vegetable rack, in front of people I had just met and would be living with for the coming year, required me to maximise my intelligence and social skills and became typical of my first year; a steep learning curve both academically and personally.

I had always wanted to become a doctor yet it was always very difficult to explain exactly why, especially on a UCAS personal statement. Whilst deciding my A level options, as well as the compulsory chemistry, my school advised me to take Maths to A2. Following my own research I added Biology, instead of Maths, as a second science. My other choices, Psychology and English literature, were a little more unusual for a budding doctor but I thoroughly enjoyed them and found that Psychology was indeed relevant during the preclinical years. My insight into the world of medicine was also enhanced when I spent time as a hospital volunteer with patients suffering from multiple sclerosis. I also shadowed a consultant physician for a week and worked part time as a hospital domestic assistant.

I decided that I would prefer an integrated course partly because of the early clinical exposure which I felt was important and also because I knew I would enjoy the variety involved – from formal lectures to early clinical visits at GP surgeries and local hospitals. Following my application I was fortunate to be invited to four interviews. I was extremely surprised at how the format of these differed. Some were extremely formal, asking me how I would run the National Health Service, probing my views on ethical issues and asking about areas of medicine with current media exposure. Others preferred to enter into a discussion about my interest in art and the philosophical aspect of colours! I eventually chose my medical school based purely upon a gut instinct when I visited the university campus.

I opted to move into a self-catering flat for my first year accommodation, which resembled a minimalist IKEA showroom. Friends I made at that time remain my best friends now. The first year started with the obligatory 'week one' which many people say is one of the best weeks they have ever experienced and mine was no different. This week consisted of having little sleep, discovering one's alcohol limit (and extending it) and learning numerous survival skills.

The transition from sixth form to degree level was difficult and I had on average 25 hours of lectures a week with reading to do on top of this in my own time. Exams were also different. A true/false examination sounded easy but I

(Continued)

(Continued.)

had never had a negatively marked exam before and this took some getting used to.

Perhaps the best and worst parts were the anatomy dissection classes. It was a privilege to be able to discover the anatomy of the human body through a weekly 3-hour group dissection of a cadaver, but it was stressful being grilled by professors at the end of each session, especially as the marks counted for the whole group, which put you under pressure not just to work for yourself but also for others.

In the latter months of the preclinical stage I undertook a dissertation, the content of which was allocated randomly. I studied the 'Notch Receptor' in rats for 4 months in a laboratory whilst others were researching more (relevant) clinical topics. However, I gained much from the experience developing skills in organisation, data analysis and literature critique and I was successful in attaining a BMedSci qualification. This was beneficial as in some other medical schools you need to take a year out to gain this qualification, instead of it being part of the 5-year course.

The Medics' social life certainly lived up to its reputation (cocktail parties, charity fundraising events, musicals, comedy nights, medical society elections, balls etc.). Everywhere I went there was a ready-made group of friends – the medics' clique. Love it or loathe it, eventually it does lure you in.

For myself the preclinical years were essentially a balancing act between the academic aspect of studying medicine, making new friends, and learning how to become independent and survive away from home. I had not expected it to be so hard to adapt initially, but after overcoming this it was packed full of fantastic memories, and confirmed to me that I definitely wanted to become a doctor.

Chapter 11 **The medical course – later years**

You have survived all the lectures, dissection, practical sessions and more importantly, numerous exams; now it is time to embark on life as a full time clinical student. It is the time to put all the theory into practice and start getting a feel for what being a doctor is really like. Life can change quite dramatically at this time. Firstly many of the students with whom you started at university will have graduated at the end of the third year. Some of these may have gained employment and be earning considerable amounts of money. As a clinical student the debts will increase further. This is not helped by the fact that holidays become scarce and it is time to buy a new wardrobe (not literally) – it is important as a clinical student to look and act the part.

There may be times as a student on the wards when you feel in the way rather than useful. The staff in a hospital will nearly always be busy and it is easy to shy away and try not to be a nuisance. This is not to be recommended. Medical students can play a very helpful role in a teaching hospital. Often you will be the first person to meet a patient when they are admitted. The impression you give initially will represent the hospital and the other staff. As a student you will often have more time to spend with the patients and through this be able to build a trust. Many of the health professionals who will see the patients later will not have the time to sit and listen as much. For this reason it is possible that you may find out information that the doctors have not elicited, and you can also follow the patient's admission more closely.

Whether in third year, fourth year or even earlier, the first real patient contact can be quite daunting. It is time to leave the jeans and T-shirts behind and completely revamp your wardrobe collection with smart outfits. Although still a student, you have a responsibility as a medic to dress and act in a professional and appropriate way. This means ironed clothes (possibly quite a shock for some people), shirts and ties. It is not necessary to go overboard – suits are not required.

11.1 Ward etiquette

As well as dressing appropriately, it is necessary to act in a manner fitting of a future doctor. Most hospitals insist on students wearing a white coat, not only to protect your own clothes but also to help prevent spread of infection. It is essential that you wear your identification badge at all times. When arriving at a ward, make yourself known to the nursing staff. Check that they don't mind you being there and ask them if any specific measures need to be taken before going to see patients. In some cases it is necessary to wear gloves and gowns etc. You must wash or sterilise your hands with alcohol gel before and after patient contact and when leaving wards. A student will normally be attached to a particular ward for a certain time, so it is worth orientating yourself early on. When approaching a patient, always introduce yourself and ask their permission before asking questions or examining them. Remember that patients will often be more scared than you are by being in hospital and for this reason you should explain clearly your examination routines or any practical procedures. In some circumstances, you may have to ask a colleague or other member of staff to act as a chaperone – if in any doubt, do not examine a patient on your own. As well as learning the skills of talking to and examining patients, you will learn practical procedures, such as taking blood. Any such procedure must be done under the supervision of a doctor in the early days – again, if in doubt, always ask a senior.

11.2 The introductory course

Before commencing the clinical course, most students embark upon an introductory lecture course. This will include presentations on:
• Taking a history from a patient
• Communication skills
• Basic examination routines
• Management of common medical and surgical conditions.
It is not possible to make this completely comprehensive within the first week – it is merely an introduction and most students will have had some experience of these concepts earlier. Taking a history is one of the main skills to be learnt initially. Doctors in all specialities use this skill, although some to a greater extent. It is the art of asking a patient questions in order to determine what is wrong with them (the *diagnosis*). Despite the wide variety of expensive tests that are available, it is often possible to make a diagnosis after asking such a history. Following on from the history, doctors tend to perform an examination. Students will learn how to perform the examination routines for various systems. It is not possible to become proficient in these new skills within the

first week but the lectures are aimed at guiding a student in the right direction. There is no substitute for actually talking to and examining as many patients as possible. A student can be shown an examination routine a thousand times in the lecture theatre but, until it is carried out personally, the skill will not be learnt.

11.3 Clinical firms

The clinical years are divided into various speciality blocks; the idea is to give you experience in most of the common specialities. Generally speaking, the more fundamental the speciality, the more time you spend studying it, but the length of each block will vary depending on the university. Traditionally a group of medical students would be attached to one particular firm – this term refers to a group of doctors of varying levels (see Chapter 15). With the advent of shift working and modernising medical careers, we have unfortunately lost this firm structure and this has had a direct effect on not only junior doctors but also medical students. This means a lack of continuity in teaching and often the loss of feeling part of a team. It is sometimes even difficult to get portfolios and log books signed by senior clinicians as often you have spent little time with them. One small advantage is that you get to experience teaching from a wider range of clinicians.

The clinical years normally commence with an introduction to medicine and surgery (junior medicine and junior surgery). During the rest of the clinical years specialities covered will include: accident and emergency, anaesthetics, dermatology, ENT (ear, nose and throat), general practice, healthcare of the elderly, obstetrics, gynaecology, ophthalmology, orthopaedics, paediatrics, psychiatry, and rheumatology. Increasingly student chosen modules are offered at some stage during the clinical years (see later section) and, of course, there is the opportunity to study medicine abroad during the elective. The majority of the fifth year concentrates on revisiting medicine and surgery at a higher level. The medicine and surgery courses cover the vast majority of the specialities under this umbrella (see the individual chapters on training in general medicine and surgery for more information on the choices). Of course, exams once again feature highly in the timetable. Please remember that the medical schools vary considerably in the timing and length of the different attachments – so check with individual institutions.

During your clinical years, you may well spend time at other hospitals around your local region. This is to ensure you experience different hospital environments (teaching versus district general) and also to prevent overcrowding: there is just not enough room in the main hospital for all the students at one

---

The clinical curriculum

- Accident and emergency
- Anaesthetics
- Dermatology
- Ear, nose and throat
- Elective
- General practice
- Healthcare of the elderly (geriatrics)
- Medicine
- Obstetrics and gynaecology

- Ophthalmology
- Orthopaedics
- Paediatrics
- Pathology
- Psychiatry
- Radiology
- Rheumatology
- Student chosen modules
- Surgery

---

time. In some instances the attachments can be 12 weeks long and up to 75 miles away. Accommodation will usually be provided by these hospitals but some people buy cars or commute and continue to live in the same place. This can be very difficult to do, especially if finances are tight, so bear it in mind for your budget.

11.4 An average week

The weekly timetables will depend on the current attachment but in general will follow a pattern. The focus of teaching will be on small group tutorials rather than large lectures, although there may be some sessions where you get together as a whole year for central themes. Many of the tutorials will now be around the bedside, learning clinical skills and practical procedures, knowledge that can be reinforced using the clinical skills and simulator laboratories. There will be timetabled teaching sessions with the more senior doctors and these could be topic or skills based. It is necessary to see patients and 'clerk' them (i.e. take a history and perform an examination), to then present to the Consultants during their ward rounds. Ad hoc teaching sessions are often as useful and can be given by the more junior staff or other healthcare professionals. Of course you need to be around on the ward for these to occur – in general the staff are too busy to be trying to track the whereabouts of the students if an opportunity for a practical procedure or interesting patient appears, so it is essential to be enthusiastic. During each attachment the relevant pathology and radiology will be taught by experts in these fields in other tutorials. Other sessions will be spent in outpatient clinics or watching procedures and operations. Not all sessions of the timetable will be structured and there will be time to spend on the wards seeing patients and improving clinical skills. It is useful during this time to see the general everyday running of the wards or GP surgeries attend the admissions wards, preferably when your Consultant is the admitting officer, and see the patients as they come into the hospital (see being 'on call'). Often the most important members of the team will be the junior doctors so tag along with them at free times. They often know where the interesting patients are and will appreciate your help with procedures such as taking blood, oh..... and they can point you in the direction of the best coffee and also the doctors mess. Our advice: be around, be enthusiastic and get involved – you will get much more out of the attachments. It is generally much easier to shy away, and to be honest this will not necessarily be noticed by medical staff, until the exams – when it is too late. Remember keen students get more teaching.

11.5 Medicine and surgery (see also Chapters 20 and 21)

Medicine and surgery are the longest components of the clinical course, and there are usually two attachments for each, junior medicine and surgery and senior medicine and surgery. The attachments can be 8–12 weeks long for each. You will spend time attached to a particular team of doctors who will supervise and teach you. There will be opportunities to see and assess patients, practise examinations, and learn clinical skills such as blood taking, resuscitation and other minor procedures. General medicine is also known as internal medicine and is discussed in more detail in Chapter 20. You will spend time on the wards, in the outpatients department, and, when studying surgery, in the operating theatre where there is the chance to assist with the operation itself. During surgery attachments many students spend the odd week learning about anaesthetics – this can be good fun and usually results in the acquisition of some useful clinical skills ranging from insertion of cannulae to intubation of patients.

11.6 Obstetrics and gynaecology

Generally, you will spend around 8 weeks in this attachment, and your time will be split between the two areas. In obstetrics, you will spend time in antenatal clinics, seeing and assessing pregnant women, and then spend time in the delivery suite helping deliver babies. This can be quite a nerve-wracking time, but do not worry; you will be closely supervised. You will also spend some time in theatre assisting with Caesarean sections. Gynaecology means time in outpatients and in theatre observing operations such as a hysterectomy.

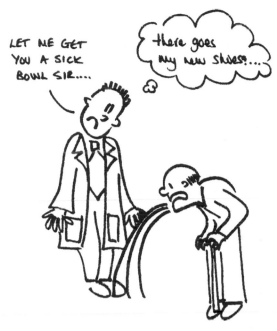

The clinical years

11.7 Paediatrics

Although it is obviously distressing seeing poorly children, most students look forward to this attachment. It involves developing different skills as the patients are often not able to give a history and it can be difficult to examine them. There is often time to be spent not only with the children but also with their playstation or other toys. It can be a difficult subject area because of the vast array of diseases that babies and children can develop. Emotions are often high and caring for and communicating with the parents is also essential.

11.8 General practice (see also Chapter 19)

The time allocated for this speciality at most universities does not correlate with the fact that the majority of graduates become GPs. Traditionally most students were only offered a small number of weeks to experience medicine at the community level. This has changed over the last few years and many students now find themselves allocated to a local GP surgery early in their course. This allows several visits over the 5 years and gives some continuity and experience of a very different kind of medicine. After all, spending so much time in the hospital, one can start to think that all patients are unwell and require emergency treatment. This is also a time when teaching is often on a one to one basis and a medical student may have there own list of patients to see. During this time it is also possible to spend time with other members of the surgery, for example district nurses, community physiotherapists. The emphasis on community care will increase over the next few years as the government moves more services out of the large acute hospitals. GP attachments should really be longer as it can be a very different kind of medicine with much less availability of instant investigations. Most students enjoy the courses where regular visits to the same surgery are organised as they appreciate the experience of continuity.

11.9 Other attachments

The attachments mentioned above tend to be the longest. The time allocated to each of the other parts of the clinical spectrum will vary. Although the specialities are divided at medical school, the reality is that there is great overlap and doctors often have joint meetings (multi-disciplinary meetings or MDTs). For example a patient with lung cancer would be discussed and seen at a clinic which could have doctors and other healthcare professionals from respiratory medicine, oncology, palliative care, radiology, pathology and thoracic surgery. In this way expertise can be offered and a management plan devised. Some subjects during the clinical years will not have an allocated time, but the relevant sections will be covered with each attachment, for example radiology and pathology i.e. the pathology and radiology of gynaecology will be studied during this attachment.

The clinical years offer an insight into the reality of becoming and working as a doctor. The attachments should be enjoyable but at the same time can be hard work. Most will have formal examinations, although some may use course work as an assessment.

11.10 On call

Another essential element of the clinical years is to spend time 'on call', preferably with members of your team. During this time it is possible to clerk (take a history and examine) many of the patients, even before the doctors have seen them. In this way a student doctor can get used to presenting the patient's history and examination findings to the more senior members of the team and also start considering management plans. It is then possible to follow the patient from their admission until their discharge. If any of the patients requires surgery or other procedures, then it is useful to attend and help at these.

11.11 Examinations and assessments

All the specialities during your clinical years will be assessed in one way or another. The timing of these will vary with each medical school. The more traditional universities favour the concept of finals. This refers to a set of examinations at the end of fifth year, which test knowledge on all the subjects studied during the clinical years. The more modern courses involve assessments at the end of blocks of subjects. This has the advantage of not revising such a huge number of subjects at the end of the course but does require more regular work throughout the clinical years. The type of examinations and assessments include those introduced in the preclinical years and also involve more practical based tests.

OSCE – Objective Structured Clinical Examination

This involves a series of stations lasting a few minutes each, where various clinical skills will be tested. This could include patient examination, taking a history, describing X-rays, or interpreting clinical data. These types of exams have been shown to be fairer because each candidate has the same questions and examiner.

OSLER – Objective Structured Long Examination Record

This assessment will probably replace the so-called long case exam. It involves a student spending a set amount of time (usually about 45 minutes) with a patient during which they take a history and perform a relevant examination. Following this they will be joined by the examiner who will ask questions about the case, which will include clinical findings, diagnosis and management. The examiners will also ask the patient's opinion of the student doctor.

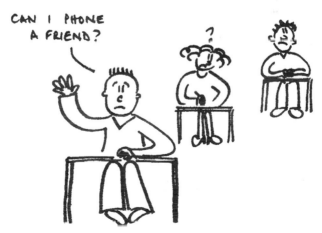

Medical examinations

Short cases

This involves a candidate seeing several cases while being accompanied by an examiner. It may involve examination of certain systems or good use of observational powers, while being questioned.

Log books and portfolios

Many of these attachments use log books as a way of assessing progression through the course. These will list objectives and then have sections to be filled in listing various practical and learning experiences that should be gained, and which need to be signed by your teachers. Not all students like the log book approach as it seems like a signature-obtaining game. It should be noted that the log books are to be used as a guide and contain the bare minimum required by a student to complete the attachment.

Student chosen modules

This concept is being introduced at an increasing number of medical schools. During the clinical years a student spends one or two clinical attachments studying a topic of their choice. This can mean further general training in paediatrics, for example, or possibly choosing a more specialist subject, which you may not experience otherwise, for example forensic medicine. The other advantage of this attachment is that there may well be no written examinations, although some course work is usually expected. If you already have an idea of your chosen speciality once you qualify, then this is a perfect opportunity to determine if your decision is correct. Bear in mind it will not be possible for every student to get their first choices. Some universities are also arranging for exchange programmes to take place in various European countries. The options will then be endless, although language may be a barrier.

The elective (see Chapter 13)

OK, so you have worked hard for the last 4 or 5 years and over the clinical years there has been little evidence of holidays. There is one part of the clinical curriculum that should be eagerly awaited – the elective. So let's get this straight: as part of your course, you are allowed to spend up to 2 months travelling the world and possibly even getting funded. Well that is not exactly true (for most at any rate!).

11.12 The shadowing weeks

A further modern concept in the medical curriculum is the introduction of the shadowing period. This will occur at the end of the course, before commencing your foundation year 1 post. The initial part of this will consist of short lectures concentrating on various practical issues, for example completing death certificates and dealing with the coroner. The majority of the time will be spent accompanying the doctor who you will be replacing in the August. This will give you the opportunity to get to know a little about the hospital where you will be starting. This is important because all hospitals differ slightly in their arrangements, for example ordering of tests. It should help you settle into what will become your new home for the next few months. It would be unwise to miss any of this time. It is your last chance to get up to speed with managing patients and procedures with maximal support from the doctors and other staff. If you feel that there are any weaknesses in the skills that you should have gained, now is the time to correct them.

11.13 Graduation

So, you have finally made it. Five years of hard work (and hopefully considerable fun) are now behind you. It is time to look forward to your chosen career and the success that this will bring. Before this, it is time for some well earned celebrating. At the end of the academic year is the formal graduation ceremony. Now is the time for the parents and loved ones to watch their children receive their graduation certificates in full gown and mortar board. They will fully appreciate the time, effort and financial support that have been necessary over the preceding 5 years. The culmination of the 5 years will be the graduation ball. No doubt, a committee will have volunteered early during the fifth year to arrange this grand event. Fund raising may actually have started many years earlier. You will only ever experience one medical graduation ball, so enjoy it!

PERSONAL VIEW   *John Findlay*

I vividly remember my first memories as a clinical student; emotionally, I would describe myself as a mix of utter excitement and, somewhat unfortunately, abject terror. Excitement, because after almost 3 years I'd thrown off the shackles of didactic lectures and learning, and was finally putting all I had learnt to practical use. Terror, because I found myself on a hectic medical ward, filled with busy staff and disconcertingly ill patients, with myself apparently utterly surplus to requirements. All of a sudden there were endless facts to assimilate, strange stethoscope noises to decipher and bewildering blood tests to interpret. To this day I have never felt more out of my depth. However, being on an 'integrated' course I had already been introduced, albeit briefly, to clinical skills which personally I found very useful. I asked a friend in the year above

(Continued)

(Continued)

whether things ever got better; he thought for a second and replied, 'not really, you just get used to feeling stupid'. Things did not bode well!

Needless to say, everything improved within days. Practice does make perfect and one of the advantages of those around you seeming to know more than yourself, is that you never stop learning! Despite the impression given by most, there are many useful tasks you can do as a medical student, and you are rarely truly surplus to requirements. The most important thing is to ask and get involved. Most doctors actually enjoy teaching, some passionately so, and these are an invaluable resource – definitely worth exploiting! It did not take long before I was feeling more confident, competent and, dare I say it, thoroughly enjoying myself. I've never looked back.

In stark contrast to preclinicals, your days on clinical attachment are extremely varied. Personally I found it quite a challenge to adapt from simply turning up to lectures every day in my casual clothes, to organising my own day balancing clinical exposure and experience with knowledge gathering from textbooks. As well as the differences you would expect between individual specialities, as a student you have a great opportunity to sample any number of experiences. Although you can easily feel like a spectator, by being proactive there is a huge amount to see and do; from being the first to take a history and examine an emergency patient, to seeing patients in clinics, or even assisting in the operating theatre. Getting the most out of your days and weeks is a vital skill. I might add that this is becoming increasingly pertinent; student intakes are escalating whilst staff are being made redundant and hence our clinical exposure is unfortunately suffering in terms of time. Whilst being a clinical student is very much as I had imagined it to be, there have been some surprises. I did not expect to be competing with my peers for diminishing access to clinics, theatres and even patients, and I was taken aback by just how much students are left to their own devices, a far cry from your spoon-fed school and early university years.

Special study modules, if offered, allow you to try something completely different (e.g. sports medicine), to revise skills and knowledge you may be lacking, or simply spend extra time studying something you enjoy. My month in anaesthetics definitely covered the latter two and allowed me to get some invaluable hands-on experience. Often as a student you have the luxury of time and can spend far longer than busy doctors and nurses with patients; sometimes this allows you to pick up previously unknown, and often important information. Other times it can give a lonely or worried person someone to talk things over with. As a student you can also lend a hand on the ward with various practical procedures such as taking blood or setting up intra-venous drips. As well as being quite fun (!) and hopefully

(Continued)

(Continued.)

helping out the other staff, it also equips you well for your future days as a junior doctor. Above all, the learning curve in medicine is really rather steep!

Of course it's not all plain sailing; there is certainly a lot of work to get under your belt, especially so if you've got distinctions or honours in your sights or finals have got you in theirs. Indeed the sheer volume to accomplish can easily become daunting. Most students find that they enjoy some attachments far more than others and if you didn't really take to a speciality, revision can be even more draining. And no matter how personable you are, your clinical skills constantly need practise and honing. There are also other hurdles to be jumped; disastrous scheduling conflicts between consultant ward rounds and the Ashes, and whether watching 'Scrubs' really qualifies as 'revision' in the true sense of the word – for what its worth, my current opinion is that it is a useful study aid! All that hard work is, however, ultimately worthwhile when you're able to diagnose and manage a patient correctly.

Another aspect to consider is that many of your friends will now be graduating, moving away and in some cases taking up rather lucrative contracts. Other friends may well be embarking on exotic holidays prior to starting work whilst you're on attachment during the summer months. All this can seem a bit unfair whilst you're still throwing money at tuition fees, textbooks, rent, student loans and the major brewing corporations. Despite this, however, your social life does not suffer too much; medics do indeed 'work hard and play hard'. Despite 'working' 47 weeks a year and some very long days, I've had the time of my life over the last couple of years. I've made some fantastic friends and even snuck in the odd adventurous holiday. I think the important thing is to find the right balance.

In summary, life as a clinical student is hard work, but for the most part great fun and in some cases extremely rewarding. I've been lucky enough to deliver babies, assist in Caesarean sections and open heart surgery, intubate and anaesthetise patients, and even diagnose a patient 15 minutes before 'Dr House' on Channel 5! I wouldn't swap it for any other course in the world.

Chapter 12 **The intercalated degree**

To *intercalate* means to insert among others, that is, the intercalated degree is one that you take during study for another.

The prime purpose of medical school is to graduate as a Bachelor of Medicine and a Bachelor of Surgery (these have various abbreviations depending on the university attended – BM BS, MB BS, MB BChir etc.). During the study for this primary degree, it is often possible to carry out some research towards an extra degree – the so-called *intercalated degree*. These vary in form – some are carried out within the 5-year medical degree course while others require extra time; some an extra 6 months, some an extra year. Most allow you to graduate as a Bachelor of Science (BSc), but there are variations on a theme.

12.1 Popularity

One-third of medical students in the UK study for an intercalated degree during their undergraduate course, but the proportion varies according to the medical school. At some schools, the opportunity to take this additional degree depends on performance in the first couple of years, whilst at others, it is an integral part of the curriculum.

12.2 The choices

There is little consistency between the types of degree offered by the different medical schools and, although some traditionally have been regarded as being better, in reality they have the same benefit. The majority of medical schools offer a BSc or a BMedSci. Occasionally the degree gained is a BA, a Bachelor of Arts degree, which is bit of a paradox considering that most medical students are very science orientated. An uncommon option that is offered is an integrated PhD. This may be done as a separate intercalated 3-year degree between

preclinical and clinical years or sometimes is integrated into an extended 5-year clinical course (for example, at Cambridge).
- BSc: available at most medical schools
- BMedSci: Nottingham, Birmingham and Newcastle
- BA: Oxford and Cambridge
- PhD: selected universities.

12.3 Which subjects are available?

The subjects are usually basic science orientated, the reason being that the departments available to join in the medical school for the projects are those teaching the basic medical sciences during the preclinical years.

Possible intercalated subjects	
• Anatomy	• Medical microbiology
• Cell biology	• Neuroscience
• Epidemiology	• Pharmacology
• History of medicine	• Physiology
• Medical biochemistry	• Psychology
• Medical law	• Public health

12.4 The objectives

The main principle behind the intercalated degree is to develop the ability to evaluate research critically and understand the principles underlying its methodology – skills necessary for life-long medical learning and practice. The best way of acquiring these analytical skills is by conducting in-depth research oneself. Also, with the deepening recruitment crisis in academic medicine, encouraging those contemplating such a career should be a priority. Thirdly, allowing medics to interact with a new and diverse peer group can broaden horizons and offer fresh perspectives on the learning process. This research period offers time to study a selected area of biomedical technology in depth, usually by means of lectures and a research project. It is hoped a student will gain:
- a greater depth of knowledge of some area of medical science that under-pins modern medicine;
- the ability to critically evaluate previous and current research, the biomedical literature and data;
- the ability to communicate scientific information in a variety of formats;

• research skills enabling design, execution, interpretation, and reporting of experiments in an area of biomedical sciences.

The experience brings some of the scientific theory learnt in the first couple of years of medical school to relevance, for example learning what PCR (polymerase chain reaction) and western blotting really are, developing good computing skills, such as database management, presentation skills, journal article searching and familiarity with statistics.

There is also a recreational element to the additional year, with more free time. This time can be spent with the many medical societies; it gives an additional extra summer with the opportunity to travel the world; and can also provide extra maturity, making you ready for the demanding clinical years.

12.5 The benefits

Educationally

If you wish to pursue an academic career, then an intercalated degree is sensible, as it will allow you to develop research skills, think critically, study the scientific basis of medical sciences and prove to others that you are academically motivated. If you really do want to work in a laboratory later in life, the experience gained during the year could be invaluable. Currently, some specialities do require that people have higher degrees, and the intercalated degree will be useful for applying for those positions. Being taught by scientific members of staff, and having the opportunity to experience the excitement and challenges of science will certainly be a change from sitting in the medical school lecture theatres.

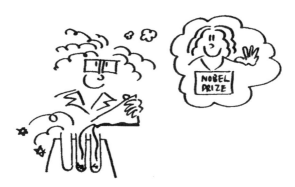

The intercalated degree

Clinically

There does not seem to be a correlation between undertaking an intercalated degree and clinical excellence. Will it help you get the best jobs when training as a junior doctor? Possibly – there is no doubt that the extra degree will look good on paper, but it is uncertain as to how much influence this would have on your chances of being shortlisted. Some of the best consultants in the country do not have an intercalated degree, indeed some of them have no formal academic research under their belt at all. Having said this, the competitive areas of medicine often use academic criteria to discriminate candidates and further higher degrees (for example, MSc, MD, PhD) can be required, and undergraduate degrees can help with securing these at a later date. Remember that, following qualification, most junior doctors' CVs are very similar, so anything that can make you stand out will be useful.

Leaving medicine

If you decide that medicine is not for you, then having a BSc or BMedSci on the CV will look good and gives you the opportunity to get out of medicine after 3 years with a recognised science degree.

12.6 The downside

Taking additional time to undertake the intercalated degree costs in terms of time and money. With medical students graduating owing over £10 000, a figure which is increasing continuously due to tuition fees and higher living costs, the additional year could be costly. Occasionally funding is available, but this is usually only available to those who are undertaking higher degrees.

12.7 It's your decision

To decide, you must weigh up the pros and cons, mainly the educational benefits versus the financial costs. One possible way round the financial costs is to plump for Nottingham or Sheffield – they offer a BMedSci without any additional year.

12.8 Other options

Another option is to complete the medical course and then take time out during your career path to study for a higher degree (MSc, MD, PhD).

PERSONAL VIEW   *Rick Harrison*

My decision to study for an intercalated degree really started before I applied to Medical School; I thought it sounded like a good idea and specifically applied to medical schools which offered the intercalated degree as part of the course. I was accepted to and chose to attend Nottingham University, which offers a BMedSci degree as part of the 5-year course. This basically means that your 'preclinical' and 'clinical' time is compressed slightly and your period of research is done during the 3rd year. It means you have to work harder than students at other medical schools, but you 'save' a year overall.

Although the intercalated degree is 'built in' at Nottingham, as with most medical schools, there was a broad choice of departments and subjects to study, for example, Pharmacology, Physiology, Anatomy. I chose the Department of Anatomy as I thought this was most relevant to what I thought I wanted to do in the future, which was Surgery.

I was allocated a supervisor who I met with on most days and he set me the research task. I had to grow cultured cells in a laboratory in different conditions to see how well they could grow. I won't blind you with the science, although it sounds 'hi-tech', all the procedures were taught to me. Friends in different departments were generally working on a small part of a large ongoing project. Some were helping out with clinical trials (those conducted on patients), some were working in the lab, whilst others were helping to write software programs. Some students even devised their own projects...

Although hard work during the day, there were no lectures to study for or tutorials to prepare for, which left the evenings free for sport or other activities, this was a pleasant break from lots of library work, which I knew would be re-starting at the end of the year.

The research project lasted for around 8 months and at the end of this, I had to complete a dissertation of around 15 000 words, which formed the basis of your assessment for the degree. This dissertation was examined with a viva exam, which was genuinely quite frightening! I was awarded a 2:1 degree which I was very pleased with.

Although hard work, I think the experience was worthwhile; medical practice is now based around research and 'evidence' and knowing how that knowledge is compiled can be very useful. Good luck if you choose to do one!

Chapter 13 **The elective**

This will become one of the most memorable parts of your medical school life. The medical elective is a period in the medical curriculum lasting between 8 and 12 weeks (depending on the individual medical school), when you are given the freedom to choose what and where you want to study. You are allowed to go to any medical establishment in the world! The major difficulties are in choosing where to go and how to afford it! Different medical schools put the elective in different places in the curriculum. It is invariably in the final 2 years of the course after you have at least some clinical training.

13.1 The official bit

The medical schools will tell you that the purpose of the elective is to allow you to explore in detail a field of medicine that you find of particular interest or an area that you felt was inadequately covered in the medical curriculum. It is included because it allows an opportunity to experience medicine in a different social, cultural, economic and scientific environment. Some medical students with a real interest in a subject, go to a renowned centre of excellence in that subject to make contacts and develop that all-important CV.

Medical schools are aware that 22-year olds given 2–3 months off might take an opportunity to have a rather good long holiday. It is therefore compulsory to write a report of what you have done, and at some universities, return a signed form from the hospital where you visited, to certify that you spent time where you said you were going to work!

13.2 The unofficial bit

Traditionally, medical students have used the elective as a once in a lifetime opportunity to travel to far flung places where the sun shines all day long and to have adventures that become the stuff of legends and the content of stories and anecdotes for the rest of their medical careers. Such as 'I was in a bar in the remotest of the Pacific islands when...?'

Most hospitals that have had medical students (especially those in traditional elective hot spots), know the score and will happily do a deal where you do so many days a week or a block of weeks to get things signed and enough information to write a report and then allow you time for travel. In this way it is possible to combine the educational and the enjoyable and keep everyone happy!

13.3 How do you choose where to go on elective?

Choosing an elective is extremely difficult. There are some fundamental questions that you need to ask yourself before you make up your mind.

What do I want to get out of my elective?

Do you want a valuable educational experience? Some people want to go to a centre of excellence for a particular discipline. If you are considering a career in a particular field it may allow you to explore this further and make some contacts for the future. This gives you an opportunity at an early stage to assess whether you really think that a particular area of medicine is for you or not. This sort of elective is more difficult to organise and can be a disappointment if things don't quite work out as you want.

If you primarily want a holiday there are lots of places that are very used to having elective students and will give you advice about where to go to explore when you get there.

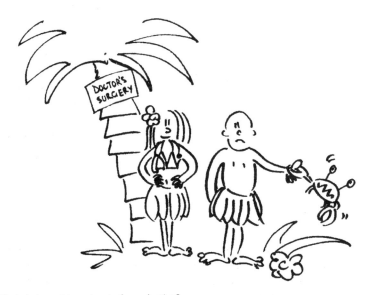

What do I want to get out of my elective?

What sort of weather do I want?

Do you want sunshine or snow? Depending on the time of year when your elect ive appears in the curriculum, you need to decide which part of the world you want to be in. If your elective is in the Autumn/Winter and you want sun then think of the southern hemisphere.

Developed or developing country?

This is a fundamental question. The practice of medicine in developing countries varies dramatically from that in the UK. The living conditions and the diseases are very different and you will see things that you may never see in the UK. Also the treatments are different and these are limited by availability of equipment, drugs, medical and nursing staff. The patients are often desperate for any medical help from anyone. In the past medical students were allowed to provide all sorts of treatment and surgery in developing countries and often benefited many patients. However you are still a medical student and as you are not qualified you shouldn't be practicing on patients in the third world. There are now strict guidelines regarding what you should and shouldn't do with regard to patient treatment on elective. Despite this you are more likely to be involved in patient care in the developing world than in developed countries.

Working in a developed country allows you to compare how medical care is organised and the good and bad points to an alternative healthcare system. However, you tend not to get as much in the way of experience.

English speaking?

You don't have to go to an English speaking country. If you have other languages then the elective is a fantastic opportunity to go and practice your language skills. If you are not very confident with another language, medical conditions and symptoms can be very confusing. The elective may allow you to develop a foreign language, but bear in mind that it is probably better to be in an environment where there is more time to talk to patients and the staff have more time to help you if your knowledge of the language is not great. For example, A&E (accident and emergency) is not a good environment for learning a new language.

Alone or with friends?

You will need to decide whether you want to go in a group or by yourself. There is safety in numbers and it does mean that you can travel with friends and remind each other of the adventures that you experienced together when you are back home. Going as a group is probably a good option if you primarily want a 'relaxing' elective.

Going as an individual will allow you to have more freedom to be who you want to be and it forces you to make more effort to meet new people. It is generally much easier to organise your elective by yourself especially if you want to go to a specific place in a specific department.

Alternatively you can try and combine it and meet up with friends on the other side of the world after your elective for a bit of travelling.

13.4 Organisation

Electives are not easy to organise from scratch. Most medical schools have copies of previous elective reports in the library with contact addresses and tips. Many consultants have colleagues/friends who work around the world. If you have a particular subject interest, then go and talk to the relevant consultants. They may be able to put you in touch with their opposite number in a foreign country. Speak with the students in the year above. Most of them will be pleased to bore you with their elective stories and you might just learn a few handy tips! Most medical schools throughout the world have a website and some have a dedicated section on electives. There are a couple of books available that give general guidance about different electives and what you can expect. However, a personal contact is the best, as there is often plenty of bureaucracy involved and if you have a friendly contact at the other end, things are much easier. Most medical schools also hold an annual elective evening with presentations from those students who went travelling the previous year, and where various travel firms are invited to have displays.

Financial limits

How much can you afford? The elective is a one off experience and it would be a shame to restrict yourself. Funding is very scarce though and will often not be available at all. Many medical schools offer small bursaries of a few hundred pounds but are only able to offer them to a small number of people. If you know what subject area interests you for your future career there are some Royal College grants and bursaries available.

Having said this, the reality is that you will probably have to fund the majority, if not all, of the elective by yourself. The BMA (British Medical Association) do offer loans at attractive rates for medical students and many think this a worthwhile thing to do. See Chapter 14 for other funding advice.

13.5 Planning

Whatever you choose you must start to plan early! Some electives are very popular, for example the flying doctors in Australia and trauma electives in

USA. If you are thinking of this sort of thing you need to start writing to the organisers about a year in advance!

Send off several applications. Reply quickly if you accept. Let people know if you decline so they can reallocate to other students. Correspondence takes time even with e-mail and there is plenty to organise other than which hospital you are going to and which consultant you will be with. You will also need to think about accommodation, necessary vaccinations, visas, medical malpractice insurance and personal health insurance.

13.6 Safety on elective

You have a responsibility to keep yourself safe on elective. Most universities can provide a travel pack with basic medical equipment and a few simple drugs (e.g. antibiotics).

Remember that HIV has a high prevalence in some countries and that precautions and even avoidance of high risk procedures is recommended.

13.7 Finally

The medical elective is a unique part of the course. Make the most of it what ever you decide to do!

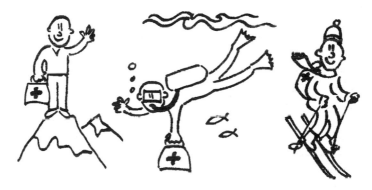

The medical elective is a unique part of the course . . . make the most of it!

PERSONAL VIEW   *Torquil Duncan-Brown*

'Here you are – you're the doctor!' These words were among the first I heard as I arrived on my student elective on the Pacific Island of Samoa. It was the senior midwife speaking and she had just deposited a blue lifeless 1 minute old

(Continued)

(Continued.)

baby into my hands. Was I petrified or exhilarated – I didn't know what to think! Here I was finally being given responsibility after all the years of learning. And what was more, I was in the most idyllic place for a hospital you can imagine. Blue skies, green seas and white beaches only a 2-minute walk away. I had got there via a week in Hawaii and was returning via New Zealand and Hong Kong.

It all needed a little organisation and planning, but I had landed myself with such a great opportunity. Not only was I going to a beautiful pacific island, but the route there enabled me to stop off and explore elsewhere. I spent the first of the 10 weeks away in Hawaii. Travellers were everywhere and I spent the week with a couple of people I met out there tripping around the islands watching sunrises from the top of a mountain, listening to whales swimming with us in the sea and drinking cocktails to the sunsets. The route back gave me the chance to see some friends for a few days in New Zealand and Hong Kong.

The work as a student in the larger of the two hospitals was a little like being at home but with my own clinics to run. When I went to the more isolated of the two islands, I found myself with more responsibility than I could have dreamed of. It all seemed a little daunting. Yet here I was running my own clinics and dealing with anything from chesty babies and children with heart failure, to pregnancies and multiple trauma casualties from car accidents. I was just entrusted to get on with it and do the best I could. I took and developed my own X-rays, did my own ward rounds and wrote prescriptions. There was always a doctor on hand to supervise, but it was an invaluable learning time when I got used to the responsibility and the chance to use all that knowledge from the past years, for what felt like the first time outside of exams. And in my spare time I got to see the tourist sites and some lesser-known places to visit on the islands. After work I would walk down to the beach and float around in the sea during the tropical storm or just relax and watch the incredible sunsets. The locals were so friendly and I became something of a local celebrity when I adopted local dress (a type of sarong) to work in! This was the life.

My elective really was one of the highlights of my student days, and looking back it has provided me with perhaps some of the vital skills for what lay ahead – my house jobs – plenty of responsibility, independence and more importantly, the ability to unwind from work.

Chapter 14 **Finances**

14.1 The hard facts

Five or six years at university doesn't come cheap. From 2006 tuition fees will be £3000 per year for all medical courses in England and Northern Ireland. There are minor variations in Wales and Scotland.

	2006–2007 (in £)	2007–2008* (in £)	2008–2009* (in £)	2009–2010* (in £)
Where in the UK?				
England	3000	3000	3000	
Wales	1200	3000	3000	
Medicine courses in Scotland	2700	2700	2700	2700
Northern Ireland	3000	3000	3000	

* The figures for these years are subject to annual increases in line with inflation.

On top of the tuition fees are considerable fees for living expenses. The loan companies anticipate that students will require about £4400 a year to cover these costs (more if in London and less if living at home). Many students find it difficult to keep within this budget. Assuming you do keep within this budget, the total cost per year (fees and living costs) will be £7400 per year which works out at £37 000 for a 5 year course. It could of course be much more.

Student outgoings

- Tuition fees
- Accommodation
- Food
- Bills
- Books/equipment
- Socialising
- Money for holidays
- Car costs/bike
- Room insurance
- Mobile phone
- Clothing
- University societies

14.2 Money management

It is important to organise your finances at the beginning of a term and try to budget for the next few weeks. Student loans are paid into your account at the beginning of term and it is necessary to avoid a false sense of wealth, otherwise you may find yourself overspent halfway through term. Many students who study medicine have affluent parents, so it is important to remember to live within your own means if your financial situation is different. Try and avoid wasting money on too many textbooks or university societies in the first few weeks. It is still possible to make purchases and join clubs later in the term. Hopefully your debt will not be too great after the first 2 years and most students manage with some common sense and knowing about certain sources of available funding.

The cheapest option at university is to live with your parents. This is not to be recommended as it is important to experience life away from home and, anyway, most students travel to a different city, so commuting is impossible. University accommodation tends to be reasonable value and the rent often covers bills and food. Once you are living away from the halls and colleges, the cost of rent is likely to increase dramatically. For popular shared houses in university towns it is not unusual to be paying around £40–60 per week, although prices can vary considerably. This does not normally include bills or food, although you won't have to pay council tax. Some areas will be more expensive than others, London being a prime example of a very expensive place.

During the clinical years it does become harder to keep your bank balance in the black. This is due to a combination of longer terms and different expenditure. Expenses include the purchase of smart clothes and possibly a car. This is obviously not essential but many of the clinical year attachments will be at other hospitals within the area, so transport is useful. Longer terms means fewer holidays and so most decide against employment and opt for exotic breaks to recover from the strenuous work.

No student should be prevented from going to university because of his or her financial situation. The Government and other organisations have methods to help those less well off. This includes help with the cost of tuition fees and also with loans. Working during a gap year can enable a few pennies to be saved ready for the start of term but most students tend to spend the money they earn during this year on travel before university. The majority of students will need to take out a student loan as a minimum. The following section covers some other sources of available income.

14.3 How am I going to pay for it?

Other than financial support from your family there are many ways to find the money to pay for your university career. The main ones are student loans, maintenance grants (for those from households with lower incomes) and awards from the university you attend. There are other separate funds available for disabled students and those with children. There are also other sources of funding such as bank loans.

Student loans

Students can now take loans for both tuition fees and living costs from the Student Loan Company (SLC) (http://www.slc.co.uk). They attract a very low rate of interest – at inflation levels. This ensures that the value of the loan that is repaid remains the same in real terms as the amount borrowed. In September 2004, the interest rate was 2.6%.

Tuition fees

From September 2006 eligible full-time undergraduate students will not have to pay tuition fees before they start university or whilst they are studying. Instead eligible students will be able to apply for a Student Loan for Fees to cover these costs (currently £3000 per annum). The fees will be paid direct to the university or college on behalf of the student. Students will repay these loans once they have left university and are earning over £15000. There are no upper age limits imposed for students' loans for fees.

Living costs

Student loans are also available to help with paying living costs. The table below shows the maximum maintenance loans available.

2006–2007	Student living at home (in £)	Student living away from home, in London (in £)	Student living away from home, outside London (in £)
Maximum full year loan rate	3415	6170	4405
Maximum final year loan rate	3085	5620	4080

The loan is repayable in instalments once you leave your course and start earning more than £15000 a year. Deductions are usually made direct from your salary (through the PAYE tax system) by your employer in the same way as tax and National Insurance contributions. Repayments are proportionate to your earnings. For example, someone earning £20000 a year would currently repay £8.65 a week or £37.50 a month. If you stop working, or your earnings fall below £15000, then you don't have to make repayments.

Maintenance grants

Eligibility for the maintenance grant depends on the household income of your family. The table below illustrates the amount and type of help that different incomes might attract. This will however vary if you study in London or live at home. The maximum grant is presently £2700. There is a variable amount of grant if the household income is between £17 500 and £37 500 a year (the table illustrates one example only). These grants will be paid at the beginning of each university term.

Annual help with living costs

Household income (in £)	17 500	26 500	37 500	50 000
Maintenance grant (in £)	2700	1200	Nil	Nil
Student loan for living costs (in £)	3200	3200	4400	3300
Total each year (in £)	5900	4400	4400	3300

If you are eligible for a maintenance grant your entitlement for a maintenance loan will be reduced by up to £1200 because the grant is paid in substitution for part of your loan.

Grants from universities and colleges

All universities running medical courses are obliged to provide non-repayable bursaries to students who are receiving the full maintenance grant (£2700). This will be at least £300 a year. Contact your university to see what they are offering.

Other grants

Some students may have specific circumstances warranting further financial help. This may come in the form of grants or allowances. As each situation is unique to the individual, it is best to make further enquiries to your LEA or contact the Department for Education and Skills (DfES).

Available grants

- NHS bursaries
- Dependant's grant
- Childcare grant
- Travel, books and equipment grant
- School meals' grant
- Lone parents' grant
- Disabled students' allowance

14.4 Other financial help available

There are other sources of funds available during term time. These are available to students having financial difficulty. It is necessary to have applied for a full student loan prior to obtaining further support.

Hardship funds

Each university has a pot of money allocated to it by the Government, which is to be distributed to those students with financial difficulties. A student loan must have been taken out and other pathways explored before applying for this fund. The amount received will depend on individual circumstances and also the number of students applying. This money does not need to be repaid.

Hardship loan

This is another loan that can be applied for if the full student loan has already been granted. The extra money is normally in the region of £500. This money will be added to your original loan account and needs repaying.

Access to Learning Fund

These funds are to help students encountering particular hardship because of a disability, living costs or childcare. The aim of the fund is to support vulnerable students, in particular to help them access and remain in higher education.

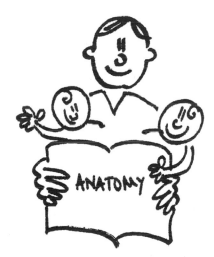

Access funds are now available for students who are parents

For example, students who meet unexpected financial crisis or who may be considering leaving their course because of financial problems. Access fund grants cannot be made for paying tuition fees.

Scholarships and awards

These are another way of funding students through university. Most institutions offer them to cover either the whole cost of the course or a contribution to it. There will be differences between the individual universities, so if you feel that extra financial help will be necessary, contact the student support centres.

14.5 Bank loans

Once the appropriate sources of income have been drained, but money is still necessary to put food on the table, it may be time to look towards a friendly bank manager. On arrival at university you should either convert your current bank account or open a new student account. A better idea would be to open a student account before arrival in your new town. During freshers' week there can be long queues at the banks. Most of the high street banks offer special introductory deals as a temptation. Study these deals carefully because, although £50 up front is a good incentive, a better interest rate on an over-draft might save you more money in the long run. There may be better deals around on the Internet but having a personal account manager at a local bank can be useful during times of trouble. Discuss the details with the individual banks to decide on which will fit your criteria the best. Most medical schools have cash machines in close proximity. Try to arrange an account manager early on.

It is fair to say that banks are especially sympathetic towards medical students. For this reason it is often possible to arrange larger overdrafts and loans than other students. This is because of the unique situation that a medical student is virtually guaranteed a job following graduation. Remember that the interest rates are not as competitive as student loans.

Pay back

As a medical student it is possible to borrow a large amount of money during university. Do not forget that this money has to be repaid at some point. The student loans company commences repayment in the April of the year following graduation. Anyone earning less than £15 000 does not need to start repayments but this will not be relevant when you are a doctor. Bank loans will be considered on an individual basis but, as the interest charges will be much higher, it is best to pay these off as quickly as possible.

14.6 Student employment

One method of preventing such a huge debt at university is to work. Many students take up holiday jobs but this becomes difficult after the third year for medical students. The other option is to actually find part-time employment in your university town. Again this can be more difficult as a medical student because of the rigours of the course, but certainly still possible. Most students opt for evening bar work or Saturday jobs.

14.7 Postgraduation

In general doctors do not tend to be the most financially astute individuals. This can be a problem if financial priorities are not realised at an early stage. As a newly qualified doctor you will be earning a significant amount of money and there is a temptation to go out and buy extravagant items. The first priority should be to pay off loans.

It is sensible to find a reliable financial advisor at this time. Be cautious in your decision because history has proven that these experts have not always been correct or indeed acted in the best interests of the individual. There are many reputable companies around and recommendation by a colleague is reassuring. Financial advisors can be independent or affiliated to one particular company. The latter can only recommend products by that one company, which can be quite limiting. The other point to check is whether you have to pay for financial advice given or if they obtain commission from the companies directly, following a policy being taken.

Postgraduation outgoings

- General Medical Council
- British Medical Association
- Medical Defence Society
- Income protection
- Postgraduate exams and courses
- Membership of postgraduate college

Wage deductions

- NHS pension contribution
- National Insurance
- Car parking
- Accommodation

Financial advisors can help with advice regarding repaying debts, pensions, saving for the future, mortgages and income protection. Income protection should be considered following graduation. Once a policy is taken out, your wage will continue to be paid if you have to have a prolonged time off work. Monthly payments are in the region of £30. Following graduation there are other compulsory payments that need to be made annually – these include membership of the General Medical Council and indemnity insurance with either the Medical Defence Union or the Medical Protection Society.

Once you are qualified you may have to complete a tax return. It is not within the remit of this book to discuss this in great detail but the following are some helpful hints.

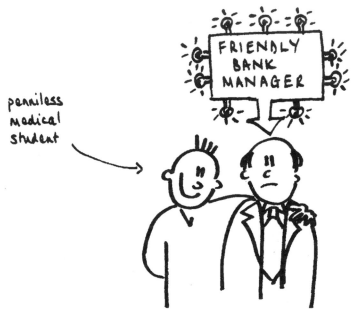

Once sources of income have been drained...it may be time to look towards a friendly bank manager

- Any income on top of your normal wage may not have been taxed at source. This includes money obtained from the completion of cremation forms.
- It is necessary to declare this extra income in order to pay the tax.

- It is wise to keep all financial documents, for example bank statements, in a safe place.
- It is possible to complete a tax return personally, but many doctors employ an accountant to do this on their behalf.

14.8 Summary

University can be expensive, but no student should be deterred from going for financial reasons. There are several available sources of finance for those struggling. The best advice is to budget carefully from the start of the term. Have an income and expenditure spreadsheet and decide how much can be spent on socialising each week. There are certain essential items, for example accommodation and food. Other items will have to be foregone if money is tight, for example mobile phone costs, alcohol, etc. Each university will be different so contact the student support groups if you think you may be in financial trouble. The earlier this is done the better, because there can be delays in the processing of forms.

We cannot recommend getting into debt up to your eyeballs, but do bear in mind that once qualified, doctors do earn a reasonable income.

Chapter 15 **House dog to top dog**

On completion of medical school, a student has reached the top of a ladder, only to then start at the base of the next one. It will take a doctor several years of training, progressing through the ranks, to be able to become an independent practitioner. This is irrespective of your final career choice, although the length of progression will depend on the speciality chosen. This chapter will describe the generic career pathway following medical school.

The medical training structure has undergone major reform in the last couple of years and this continues to be the case. Many of the possible changes proposed in the first edition of this book are now mandatory. We will describe the old system first and then the outlined structure in the new proposals. Despite the fact that the new structure will be in place by August 2007,

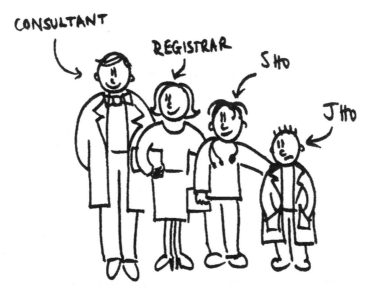

Teams of doctors in hospitals are referred to as firms

there is still much uncertainty. The changes are being overseen by the Modernising Medical Careers group and for the most up to date information we recommend reviewing their website www.mmc.nhs.uk. Another essential read is the British Medical Association website, which has information for all levels of students and doctors, with important documents updated annually (www.bma.org.uk).

15.1 The old system

Figure 15.1 summarises how a doctor's career used to progress, irrespective of particular specialisation. Following graduation a medical student became a Pre-Registration House Officer (PRHO, previously known as a Junior House Officer (JHO), or more affectionately as House Officer, House Plant or House Dog!). Pre-registration basically reflected the fact that newly qualified

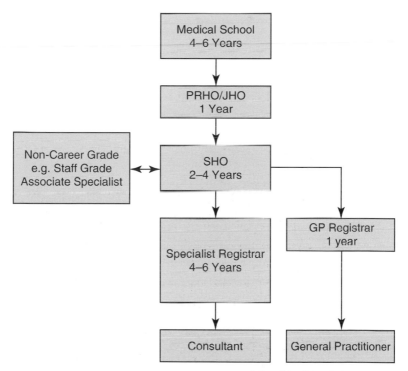

Figure 15.1 Simplified diagrammatic representation of the old training ladder for doctors – see text for details.

doctors are granted provisional registration with the General Medical Council. This position was for 12 months and usually consisted of two (or occasionally three) rotations at a couple of different hospitals. The rotations were generally divided into 6 months of medical jobs and then 6 months of surgical positions. If a doctor was successful at completing the first year, they could then fully register with the GMC (General Medical Council) and apply for their next post which would be at Senior House Officer (SHO) level. The SHO jobs could either be stand-alone 6 month positions (e.g. accident and emergency), or a doctor could enter a 2 or 3 year 'rotation' in a chosen field i.e. medicine, surgery, paediatrics (see Chapter 18 – Career Options). Many doctors also spent time working abroad during their early years. Following the completion of a speciality SHO rotation and postgraduate exams, a doctor could then apply to become a specialist registrar (SpR) in one particular area of their chosen field (e.g. SpR in cardiology, chosen field would have been medicine). Doctors training to become general practitioners would complete 2 years as an SHO and 1 year as a GP registrar and would then be eligible to be independent practitioners. SpR training usually lasted between 4 and6 years and could include further examinations. Once complete, a doctor would be eligible to gain a Certificate of Completion of Specialist Training (CCST) and become a Consultant.

15.2 Modernising medical careers (MMC)

Over the last 10 years, attempts have been made to change medical training for the better. The introduction of the PRHO year and the SpR grade following the Calman report in 1993 made some improvements. There was still the problem at the SHO level with wide variety in the quality and consistency of jobs. There was no clear career pathway and continued problems between training and service commitment. The MMC was devised to help streamline this training of junior doctors from graduation up to the point of independent practice. The main difference between the systems will be that progress through training will no longer be determined by experience and knowledge but by evidence of the outcomes of training, demonstrated through competency-based assessment. The aim is to implement focused, streamlined training for all grades. In principle this should mean better training, more supervision, increased flexibility and defined competencies to be gained before progression to the next level. The reality is yet to be seen but will certainly mean increased paper work (more ticking boxes), continued assessments and probably a less experienced work force in more senior positions. Another draw back is that there could well be doctors facing unemployment in the future – making the profession even more competitive.

15.3 The Foundation Programme

During their final year, medical students will apply for a place on a foundation programme. This is a 2-year programme of general training which was implemented in August 2005 and has been introduced to form a bridge between medical school and specialist/general practice training. Over the 2 years a doctor will rotate through a number of specialities in various health care settings. Rather than just experiencing general medicine and surgery, the foundation programme will allow a greater choice of attachments e.g. anaesthetics, general practice or psychiatry. This enables greater experience at an earlier stage which could help with future career decisions. The placements will each last 4 months, which potentially means some time could be spent in up to eight specialities. Emphasis will still be placed on the importance of medicine and surgery, so most programmes will include two medical and surgical jobs. The postgraduate training involved in the foundation programme is organised locally by the postgraduate deanery and will be administered through the so-called 'foundation schools'. These schools will consist of medical schools, local deaneries and other health care providers such as the acute hospitals, primary care trusts and organisations such as hospices. This will enable an increased variety of specialities and also settings in which to work e.g. acute hospitals, the community, mental health and general practice. There are 26 foundation schools as of 2006, with each being responsible for around 300 doctors.

With the introduction of this new programme, there has also been a change in the format of application for jobs. Previously each university was affiliated with enough PRHO placements for the number of graduates. The majority of the posts were located in the same geographic region and each student applied to a local computer matching scheme with their preferences. The application system has now completely changed with a new national online service called Medical Training Application Service (MTAS – www.mtas.nhs.uk). All medical students have to apply using this online application form and will be required to rank their foundation school choices in order of preference. Details of all the rotations will be available on the website, which at the time of writing is still under construction. Following the application, an overall score will be given to each candidate which will comprise an academic score provided by their medical school and a score relating to their application answers. It is anticipated that the closing date for applications will be during the December of the fifth year. Interviews are not likely to be part of the matching process. If a candidate does not get their first choice foundation school, their documentation is automatically forwarded to their next ranked choice of school. This process may be repeated until all available places are filled. Graduates will then be matched to a 2-year foundation programme, attracting a 2-year contract of employment.

The first year of the Foundation Programme (Foundation Year 1 – FY1 or F1), is similar to the old PRHO year, building on the knowledge, skills and competencies acquired during university. Instead of two 6-month placements, this year will be divided into 4-month attachments. The GMC, along with the local postgraduate deanery, will be responsible for this stage of training and F1 trainees will need to demonstrate areas of competence outlined in the GMC's 'the new doctor' in order to be recommended for full registration at the end of the first year.

The first Foundation year 2 (FY2 or F2) programmes began in August 2006. The F2 year will equate with SHO year 1 but, again, the jobs will consist of 3, 4-month placements. The PMETB (Postgraduate Medical Education and Training Board), along with the deanery, has responsibility for postgraduate training from this year onwards. The emphasis during this second year is again on achieving core competencies as outlined in the joint MMC/Academy of Medical Royal Colleges curriculum. This will build on the skills developed during the first year and also concentrate on other more generic issues such as team working, communication skills and use of evidence based medicine.

To summarise, Foundation programmes should, within a structured programme, deliver training in the broad, generic competencies that every doctor will need during his/her career. They are designed to give trainees the opportunity to experience a range of clinical settings. Both F1 and F2 trainees will need to provide evidence that the competencies outlined in the curriculum have been achieved and this will be helped by developing a training portfolio and using newly introduced assessment tools where doctors' skills are directly observed. Each doctor is allocated an Educational Supervisor who will be a senior clinician, not directly working with the trainee. They will organise regular meetings to review the progress and run through an appraisal process. The training portfolio will be used at these meetings to check the doctor is progressing appropriately. Each doctor also has their own consultant to assist in their progression and during the year will have a couple of review meetings with the foundation programme director (another senior consultant). This director is responsible for signing a trainee off, to enable them to progress to the next stage of training. If adequate competencies have not been achieved then a doctor may need to repeat all or some of the year. In principle these changes would seem to be for the better, but the reality is currently unclear – spending less time in more jobs could actually equate to doctors being less experienced at the basics!

Advantages to the Foundation Programme

• Trainee centred
• Single UK curriculum defining training over the 2 years

- Nationally agreed training portfolio
- Named educational supervisor
- Regular reviews and appraisals
- Increased variety of placements
- Competency based assessments
- Single application process
- Increased supervision initially.

Disadvantages to the Foundation Programme

- National application process
- More paperwork and ticking boxes
- Less time in each post
- More supernumerary positions
- Less experienced at the end due to shorter hours
- Increased supervision.

15.4 Specialist Training (ST)

Following completion of the Foundation Programme, doctors will apply for Specialist Training (ST) programmes (hospital specialities or general practice) also known as 'run-through training'. Evidence of completion of the Foundation programme will be necessary and then a doctor can apply, to what will again be a centralised national application, online (MTAS). This will be a competitive process and those successful can then continue their training to hopefully gain a Certificate of Completion of Training (CCT), following which they will be able to work independently. The ST years will involve a new integrated and streamlined training combining the previous SHO and SpR grades in to one so-called run-through grade. The main reason for this change was the lack of structure to the SHO grade. The aim now is to have a well organised and structured programme with a clear curriculum within a seamless training process incorporating both the grades. Progress throughout the programme will be through competency based assessment (in a similar way to the Foundation Programme). These curricula are being developed and overseen by the PMETB and the medical Royal Colleges. The programmes and length of training will vary with each speciality and the specifics have yet to be finalised as this book goes to press. What is known is that the programmes will initially be broad-based with increased specialisation as a trainee progresses. After completion of an ST programme, a doctor will be legally eligible for entry to the Specialist or GP register and can then apply for an appropriate senior medical appointment. Figure 15.2 summarises the modernising medical careers framework.

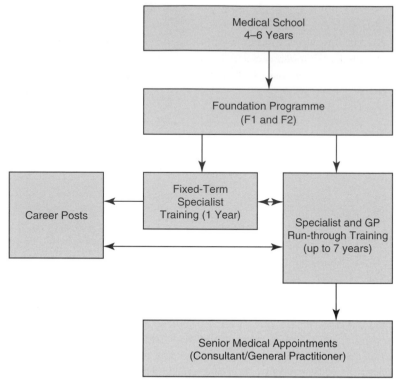

Figure 15.2 Simplified diagrammatic representation of the proposed generic training ladder for doctors – see text for details.

15.5 Fixed-Term Specialist Training and Career Posts

Fixed-term ST posts are 1-year appointments in a given speciality. The training will be the same as for a trainee in the run-through programme without the progression. The options after this year will be to apply for an appropriate ST post and hence get back on the run-through training ladder, or apply for a career post in the appropriate speciality. The career posts are service delivery positions meaning there is no formalised speciality training elements (similar to the old staff grade appointments). Emphasis will still be placed on regular appraisal and continuing professional development. The posts are only available in secondary care and a doctor will need to have completed at least 3 years of post-registration training before taking on such an appointment. Figure 15.2

shows in more detail where these posts fit in to the modernising medical careers framework. The career posts will be an equivalent of the current staff grade and associate specialist group of doctors. These are positions that can be taken if a doctor does not wish to become a consultant or is unable to do so. Several years experience in the hospital speciality is necessary, but these posts do not require a doctor to be on the specialist register and for this reason they are responsible to a named consultant and hence not completely independent practitioners.

15.6 Advantages of the ST programmes

- Seamless progression from foundation programmes to ST
- Broadly-based speciality training at first, progressing to greater specialisation
- Flexibility if career aspirations change, with recognition of previous experience
- Rigorous in-training assessment
- Flexibility to allow the pursuit of academia, out-of-programme experience and the opportunity to train less than full time
- Good career counselling and efficient manpower planning.

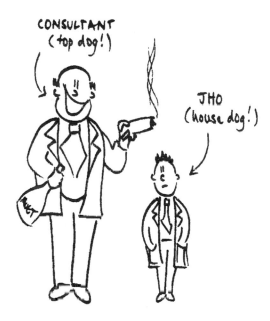

15.7 Possible disadvantages of the ST programmes

• Lack of training positions compared to number to doctors
• Producing less experienced consultants
• National, centralised online application process leading to less personalisation
• The introduction of a new sub-consultant grade
• More difficult to work abroad.

15.8 Senior medical appointments

Once the run-through training has been completed and a CCT has been awarded, a doctor is eligible to apply for a senior medical appointment. These positions include GP principals, consultants and other employed GPs. This means that a doctor is qualified to practice independently and with that has the ultimate responsibility for the patients under their care (the Top Dog!). Once a doctor has reached the level of Consultant they may also carry out private work in addition to their NHS commitments.

PERSONAL VIEW   *Bryony Elliott*

I am writing this vignette as a PRHO 6 months out of Nottingham medical school. I am one of many doctors in the first 'guinea pig' year of the Foundation Programme.

   As with every new system there have been surprising developments along the way. During the application process there did not seem to be a long term itinerary for when things would happen, or indeed how. It all seemed to be a case of trial and error. Thankfully the Trent deanery pushed the boat out and organised 2-year rotations where other deaneries throughout the country were only organising F1 posts. This allowed me and many of my peers to plan the next 2 years of our lives. The process started with a complicated online application form. We had to give evidence of situations in which we had shown particular characteristics, list fourth year examination grades and provide details of two referees. Along with this we had to rank our choice of jobs. Individuals had to decide where they wanted to work and which jobs incorporated the specialities they wanted to experience. We were then ranked, based on our application forms and matched to our choice of jobs, by what felt like a completely random process. The majority of my friends did well. The deanery reported that about 70% of my year got one of their top three jobs. However I had friends who for no apparent reason did not get matched and had to go through an

(Continued)

(Continued)

extra clearing stage. It never became clear why they were so unlucky, and they certainly never got feedback on which part of the application had let them down.

Happily I got my first ranked job, and am currently on a 2-year rotation which will include general medicine, urology, general practice, cardiology, obstetrics and gynaecology, and trauma and orthopaedics. I consider myself lucky that I will be able to experience all these specialities before choosing which path I want to take, because like a lot of people I still don't have a clue where I want to end up! This seems much more satisfying than the old system during which I would have done 6 months of medicine and 6 months of surgery, and then had to decide on my career path. On the flip side, however, there are some people in my year who are certain about their career path. They feel that they are just passing time in different specialities waiting to apply for the speciality training programme of their choice. And similarly there is a question whether people who have had experience of a speciality in their Foundation Programme will be looked upon more favourably in the application process for speciality training. This seems a little unfair on people who did not get a foundation programme with a particular speciality or for those who have had a change of heart on the career front.

My day to day job is much like it would have been in the old system, and in my view a vital part of the development of any junior doctor. I provide a service, which is like being the ward dogs' body. It certainly lacks the glamour of ER (emergency room)! I take blood, chase the results and make sure the results of scans and tests are in the notes ready for more senior review. However, it is in my power to make a big difference to patient care. With no clinic or theatre commitments it is the F1 trainees who have the time to talk to patients and their families. At the heart of it the F1 trainee is on the ground as the first port of call, dealing with patients. If the nurses are worried about someone they call the junior doctor, and it is this exposure to acutely unwell patients that improves your clinical and diagnostic skills.

As a foundation programme trainee I have been allocated an educational supervisor (someone independent to my working team) to help me keep track of my long term aims and progress, and a clinical supervisor (my consultant) who gives feedback on my working practice. There are timetabled meetings throughout the year at which we have to document our discussions and plan further appointments. In my opinion this has been valuable and a welcome development in junior doctor training. I feel like I have a structured support network of people who I can turn to for support, and perhaps more importantly advice about where my career is going from here.

(Continued)

(*Continued.*)

As part of the training I have to keep a portfolio, much like the RITA (Record of In Training Assessment) kept by more senior doctors. This is evidence of procedures I have carried out and experience I have gained. There are set aims and objectives that all training schemes nationwide have to adhere to. In reality this means I have protected 1-hour teaching sessions once a week, during which the Trust supplies teaching on core topics in the curriculum. The theory is that by the end of both the F1, and then the F2 years, each and every doctor will have completed the core competencies before moving on to further training. These competencies are tested by a variety of assessments, from peer review tools to direct observation in a clinical setting. Trainees are also encouraged to actively reflect on their practise and how they have dealt with certain situations. The idea is that doctors are being encouraged to recognise their strengths and weaknesses and identify areas for improvement.

I have really enjoyed working life so far. As a student I used to feel that I got in the way and it is great to finally have a role. I do sometimes feel like a small cog in a very large machine, and it is easy to think that the mundane administrative tasks are unimportant. But then I remind myself that if I did not fill in the form and take it to the radiologists, my patient would not get the necessary scan, and their diagnosis would be delayed. Working for the NHS involves being part of a massive team. I have met hundreds of people since I have started working and the people I work with have been a big part of my life. The majority of the F1 trainees live in hospital accommodation and there is a great camaraderie and an active social life. I am excited by the chance to experience a diverse range of specialities in the next two years, and hopefully somewhere along the line I will come up with a plan for the future.

Chapter 16 **Working patterns and wages**

16.1 Recent changes

Before discussing the various working patterns and pay schemes for junior doctors, it is necessary to mention some of the changes seen within the health service over the last few years. Until fairly recently it was not uncommon for a junior doctor to be working over 100 hours in a single week. Research has shown that tired doctors do not function to the best of their abilities. There can be an effect on a doctor's performance, which can lead to safety issues for the patients, but there can also be direct effects on the health and wellbeing of the individual doctor. This can then escalate and lead to problems with social and family life. By the 1990s these potential problems had been realised, and it was decided that regulations should be imposed on the maximum number of hours that doctors should be working in a week. The reduction in hours also meant that there needed to be a change in working patterns. More information and up to date guidance on hours and wages can be found on the BMA (British Medical Association) website and by reading the BMA's *Junior Doctors' Handbook*.

16.2 The New Deal

Owing to the great concern about the long hours that junior doctors were working, the Government, NHS personnel and doctor representatives agreed, in 1991, on a new working practice for training doctors. This was called *Junior Doctors – The New Deal*. As well as trying to reduce the number of hours, this document also aimed to improve such issues as doctors' accommodation and provision of food within the hospital out of hours. Until this time, shift work was rare and the majority of doctors were working on-call rosters. The New Deal suggested that the introduction of shift patterns could help reduce the number of hours worked (the types of rota are discussed in the next section). By the end of 1996, the maximum number of hours worked per week for each different type of shift had been decided. These were 72 hours for on call,

64 hours for partial shift and 56 hours for full shift. As well as this, it was decided that the average working week over the full contract of the job should average out at no more than 56 hours per week.

The New Deal hours implementation

- *1994* No doctor should be working more than 56 hours (on average) per week
- *1996* Maximum hours per week for the different shifts implemented (e.g. 72 hours for on-call pattern)
- *2000* Actual *contractual* requirement for limits on hours
- *2001* *All* New Deal hour limits and rest requirements contractual for Pre-Registration House Officer (PRHO) grade
- *2003* As 2001 but for *all* other training doctors

Unfortunately, although the Government advised this legislation, hospitals in general were extremely slow to implement any changes. Even by 2002 almost one-third of junior doctors were still working outside the New Deal limits. To improve this situation, further measures were taken in 2000 as part of the new Junior Doctor Contract, which was negotiated by the Junior Doctors Committee (JDC). This stated that the New Deal hours per week and rest requirements would become a contractual obligation for a hospital when new doctors were employed. This meant that in essence it would be illegal for a hospital to employ a doctor on a contract that was outside the New Deal guidelines. The deadline for PRHO posts was August 2001 and for other training doctors August 2003. To determine the actual number of hours worked in a week, it is necessary for the junior doctors to monitor their hours – this is also a contractual obligation. If they are found to be outside the New Deal target, hospital trusts are at risk of losing recognition for the posts (that is they risk losing the doctors).

16.3 Junior doctor working patterns

There are different types of rotas currently used by hospitals for junior doctors. This will not only depend on which hospital you work at but also the speciality you have chosen.

On call

Historically, most training doctors, regardless of speciality, worked this rota. For this pattern, a doctor would work a normal 0900–1700 day, followed by an on-call period from 1700 until 0900 the next morning and then another normal 0900–1700 day (a total of 32 hours). During the on-call period, it would be expected that a doctor would be actually working only for half of this time, the rest of the time being spent resting, preferably with some sleep (that is at least 8 hours rest) – in reality, the on-call for many jobs is actually busier than the normal working day. This rota could also include working at the weekend: a doctor would work Saturday morning until Monday evening (a total of 56 hours).

Partial shift

These rotas became more common towards the late 1990s. Doctors will work a combination of shifts to cover the emergency work but the majority of their time should be spent within working hours, i.e. 0900–1700. The maximum shift length should be 16 hours with 4 hours rest during the period. With this shift pattern doctors will take it in turns to work night shifts and when working at night, have the following day to sleep.

Full shift

These shifts are commonly used in other professions. In medicine the most common speciality to use a full shift pattern is A&E (accident and emergency). The whole rota is of a shift variety with no routine 0900–1700 days. The maximum time allowed to work each shift is 14 hours although most shifts will be between 8 and 12 hours.

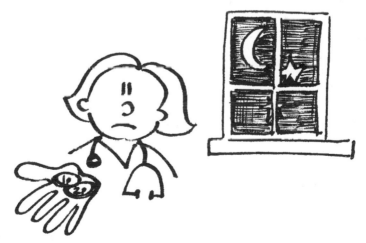

which meant that a doctor would earn a third of her normal wage when working on call

Hybrid rota

This is a combination of the above.

Working pattern	Maximum continuous period of duty (hours)	Minimum period off between duties (hours)	Minimum rest during the duty
Full shift	14	8	Natural breaks
Partial shift	16	8	¼ out-of-hours duty
On call	32 (56 at weekend)	12	½ out-of-hours duty

16.4 The European Working Time Directive (EWTD)

This directive is European law and was introduced to protect the health and safety of all workers within the European Union (not just doctors). It was introduced in 1998 but initially junior doctors were not included. After discussions in 2000, it was decided that the new legislation would affect junior doctors and that the changes would be incorporated over the next 9–11 years. The main effects on working hours are summarised below.

European Working Time Directive timetable

August 2004
• 58 hour maximum working week
• Rest and break requirements enforced

August 2007
• 56 hour maximum working week

August 2009
• 48 hour maximum working week
• Possibly extended to 2012 with 52 hour week in 2009

The changes in rest requirements become compulsory in 2004 and have been summarised below.

European Working Time Directive rest requirements (by 2004)

• Minimum daily consecutive rest period of 11 hours
• Minimum rest period of 24 hours in each 7 day period or 48 hours in 14 days
• Minimum rest break of 20 minutes if shift exceeds 6 hours
• Minimum 4 weeks of paid annual leave
• All hours spent at hospital counted as actual work
• Maximum of 8 hours work in any 24 hours for night workers in stressful jobs

---

16.5 The new pay system

The traditional pay system for junior doctors consisted of a basic salary, which would cover the normal working day, and then an hourly rate for time spent on call which was classed as additional duty hours (ADHs). The ADHs were divided into categories depending on the intensity of the work out of hours. Most jobs were defined as being class 3, which in real terms meant a doctor would earn a third of his normal wage when working on call. This should have represented the fact that the doctor would only *actually* be working for a third of the time (that is 8 hours rest in a 24-hour period). Unfortunately, as discussed earlier, the intensity of many jobs was such that very little rest was obtained – in summary, a fairly poor deal.

December 2000 saw the end of ADHs and the introduction of a new banding system. The basic salary remains the same but now a doctor will receive a supplemental payment corresponding to the amount of out-of-hours work performed. The supplement is calculated as a proportion of the basic salary and depends on the working pattern, total hours worked and the antisocial nature of a post. Those posts with longer and more antisocial hours are rewarded with a greater supplement.

The new system is divided into four bands (there are further subdivisions of Bands 1 and 2 depending on actual intensity of the job).

The banding levels

Band 3
• All doctors whose jobs are non-compliant with the New Deal (see above)
Band 2
• Jobs compliant with the New Deal and working over 48 hours but less than 56 hours per week
Band 1
• Jobs compliant with the New Deal and working less than 48 hours per week
Band F
• Jobs less than 40 hours per week

Financially it is obviously much better to be working a job with a Band 3 wage but socially not so! Unfortunately, these jobs are not compliant with the New Deal or EWTD and so are in essence illegal. There have been virtually no jobs paid at Band 3 since 2005 and with the current financial climate most hospitals have now devised compliant rotas, so most doctors are on Band 1. It is recommended to keep abreast of developments and, if you are in doubt, contact the BMA.

16.6 Is change for the better?

Surely, reducing the number of hours that a junior doctor works has to be an advantage for those who will be graduating in the not-too-distant future. From the surface it would seem that fewer hours and more pay is a great idea. Certainly patient safety is of paramount importance and it has been shown that a tired doctor could risk making more mistakes. As well as patient safety,

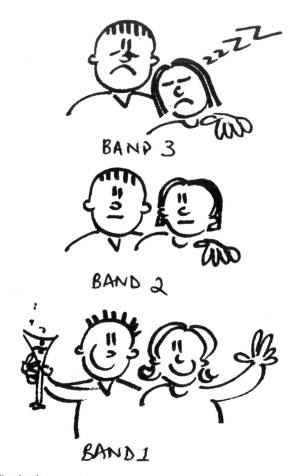

The banding levels

other advantages include the positive effect working fewer hours should have on the health and wellbeing of a doctor. This in turn should lead to better enjoyment of family and social life.

It is important to look at the argument from different angles and realise that the grass may not necessarily be greener. The main disadvantage will be the loss of the traditional firm structure for teams of doctors. Consequently there will be disruption to the continuity of care of patients and the disadvantages that this may bring. Already we are seeing patients who change wards while they are in hospital and sometimes see a different doctor each day – not good for the patient or the doctor, who then has to start from scratch and determine the correct diagnosis and which tests have already been performed. The other real worry is that, if the number of hours a doctor works in a week is cut, surely the actual length of training they receive should increase? Certainly for surgery a patient needs a doctor who has spent the relevant time cutting in the operating theatre, rather than spending many nights on call gaining little experience. The response to this is that other countries (for example, in Europe and Australia) have much shorter training programmes with no ill effect on the quality of the doctors produced. It is also felt that, if a doctor is less tired, then it is possible to get quality training in a shorter period of time. One other disadvantage is that although the total number of hours will be reduced, full shift rotas often mean an increase in the amount of anti-social hours worked.

The current reality is that doctors often find themselves working in different teams each time they are at work and patients are often unsure who their actual doctors are – neither satisfactory. With the reduction in hours, the experience of junior doctors is also being reduced which can lead to increased pressure on the more senior doctors and with the government wanting to lower the total number of years of training we may end up with less experienced senior doctors running the show!

> **Disadvantages to shift working**
> - Loss of patient continuity
> - Working more weekends
> - Reduced exposure to clinical conditions
> - Possible training opportunities missed
> - Fewer hours in the week for learning skills
> - Loss of the hospital firm structure of doctors

Lying about the amount of hours and intensity of work is not to be encouraged. This was fairly common during the early days of banding, to try and avoid the move to shift pattern rotas. Most doctors now realise that the change to shifts is not optional so this practice is ending. One other slight irony is that a doctor may well end up working more weekends with the new system. Previously many doctors would be working a one-in-four on-call rota (meaning every fourth night or fourth weekend they would be on call). The New Deal will mean on-call rotas will become a thing of the past: with the same number of doctors it would be necessary to work one in two weekends but only for certain shifts, for example 0900–2100 (that is, two 12-hour shifts, rather than working the full 56 hours). This situation should improve as the number of doctors increases.

Some doctors do not want to cut their hours down and do believe that training will suffer. However, the days for arguing are over and there is nothing the union representatives can do because the New Deal and European Directive are now law.

The best advice is to research thoroughly the jobs that you are applying for and check through the contracts carefully before signing them. If in any doubt then contact the BMA.

16.7 Flexible training in hospital

Another recent improvement has been the awareness of an increased need for flexible training. This enables doctors to work less than full time but still in posts that are recognised and count towards training. Traditionally this has been useful for those doctors with family commitments and in general the opportunities have been taken by many mothers. More recently individuals with other reasons have decided to train flexibly (see 'Personal view') and consideration will be taken if a doctor has 'well-founded individual reasons'. These can include sporting commitments, family life and problems with ill health. The possibility of flexible training and the number of flexible years allowed depend on the speciality and some of the training time may need to be full time. An applicant needs to discuss the possibility of flexible training with the relevant postgraduate deanery. There are 3 options for flexible training: slot share, job share and supernumerary. Slot share is where 2 doctors share a post, working approx 60% each so there is overlap which is useful for continuity. Job share posts are not encouraged and literally mean 2 doctors work 50% each of one post. Supernumerary posts are when a doctor is training in addition to the number of required trainees and there is a lack of another suitable flexible trainee and so slot share is not possible.

Doctors who take up GP positions often find flexible training easier and this is certainly the case as a salaried GP (see Chapter 19 for more information).

16.8 The loot

So 5 years at university and up to £20 000 of debt – is it all worth it and more to the point, how long until that Porsche purchase. Doctors earn a comfortable salary but few will become mega-earners. Financial gain is certainly not a reason for becoming a doctor especially as it could take several years to pay off all the debts. Some GPs can earn in excess of hospital consultants, but private practice in certain specialities can be lucrative (e.g. surgery). In general the wages reflect the responsibility and hence there is an increase as a doctor becomes more senior. Table 16.1 summarises some of the pay scales. These are the basic salaries and do not incorporate the banding supplements. The banding supplement can be calculated by the following: Band 1C 20%, Band 1B 40%, Band 1A and 2B 50%, Band 2A 80% and Band 3 100% e.g. if a doctor was earning £20 000 basic in a Band 3 post, their actual wage would be £40 000. Consultants' wages are more complicated, and in general higher than the table suggests because over time they earn additional supplements e.g. clinical excellence, discretionary points and distinction awards. The figures are also from the old contract. The final salary of a partnered GP will depend on the income of the whole practice.

Table 16.1 Basic salaries as at 2005

Grade	Minimum wage (£)	Maximum (£)
PRHO/F1	20 741	23 411
SHO/F2	25 882	36 292
SpR	28 930	43 931
Consultant (Old Contract)	57 944	75 404

PERSONAL VIEW   *Tim Brabants*

From first gaining a place at Nottingham University Medical School I knew my career path was likely to be a little unconventional. I was heavily involved in the sport of sprint kayak racing and knew this was something I wanted to continue in parallel with medical training. Nottingham was really my only choice of university as it has the National Watersport's centre and a good kayak club locally. The difficulty is that training for my sport requires around 14 sessions per week, either on the water, in the gym, running, swimming or cycling and on top of this were winter training camps abroad and racing trips during the summer.

(Continued)

(Continued)

In 1996 when I started medical school I had just missed out qualifying for the Olympic Games. The first 2 years at university taught me even more about time management trying to fit in training before and after lectures as well as finding time to study and pass exams. Social life took a massive back seat! The long holiday periods enabled me to go abroad on the training camps and I could fit in the racing trips with minimal disruption. The difficulty came in the third year when holiday times were reduced and this coincided with the Olympic qualifying year. I managed to keep on top of passing exams whilst training hard. My medical student housemates were essential in this process as they always made sure I knew when deadlines were and put up with my constant tiredness and occasional grumpiness!

After qualifying for the Sydney Olympics in the summer of 1999 I had the problem of how was I going to manage the fourth year with only 4 weeks off over the whole year. Luckily the Dean at the time was very keen on sports and agreed to allow me to split my fourth year over 2 years. This allowed 3 months off over the winter to spend away warm weather training, then 6 months off over the build up to the Games and time off after. This flexibility proved invaluable when I came home from Sydney with a bronze medal – Britain's first ever Olympic medal in sprint kayaking history.

It was rather strange after all the post Olympic hype and media coverage to then return to medical school in the year below, not knowing anyone, but most people knowing who I was! I made new friends and with continued support from them I was successful in completing the final 18 months of medical school and ending up graduating in the summer of 2002. I also become European Champion in the same year.

Fortunately the NHS flexible careers scheme was just being started as I graduated. Nottingham City hospital took me on to work as a PRHO one day a week for the next 2 years in the build up to the Athens Olympics in 2004. This was an excellent opportunity to keep my hand in on the medical side of things and increase the volume of training for my sport. If I went away on a training camp, I could make up the work missed by working 2 days a week for a while. The flexibility was excellent and I was basically an extra pair of hands on either the surgical or medical assessment units, normally on Mondays, the busiest day.

My second Olympics was a little disappointing. I broke the world record in the heat but only managed fifth place in the final. After that my career took priority for the first time in 8 years! I became a full time PRHO in Nottingham for a year in order to gain full registration with the General Medical Council. Following this I moved to Jersey for a 6 month A&E post as a SHO, with the aim

(Continued)

(Continued.)

of gaining further experience to enable me to do some locum work when yes, I went back to paddling full time!

I now work very little, train a lot and became European Champion again after 5 months back to full time sport. I'm going faster than ever and think working full time for 18 months was actually the rest my body needed! I've loved my unconventional career path and couldn't have done it without the support from many people. Beijing Olympics in 2008 is the next plan, then it really is retirement from that level of competition. Most of the people I started medical school with are now taking up registrar posts and doing really well, I'll catch up eventually!

Chapter 17 **Life as a doctor**

Five years of hard graft and multiple examinations and you finally have the honour of changing all your bank cards so that they read Dr! Some may say this is pretentious but most would think you have deserved it. Has the previous 5 years fully prepared you for the next few months of your life? Although you will have gained theoretical knowledge, you will still be lacking the practical skills and experience to be fully confident in your new job. Reading about and understanding an illness in a book is very different to seeing it in real life, especially if the patient is acutely unwell. Most graduates do find the transition from medical student to qualified doctor difficult – do not worry – all junior doctors have been through this and most have continued in their chosen career.

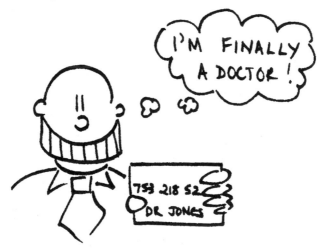

You may have the honour of changing all your bank cards so that they read Dr!

17.1 The Foundation Year One (F1, FY1)

Following graduation a medical student becomes a Foundation Year One doctor. Prior to the introduction of the foundation programme, this first year was known as the Pre-Registration House Officer (PRHO) year (or Junior House Officer (JHO)). It is a common misconception that the term junior doctor refers only to your first year following graduation. A junior doctor is in fact any doctor in a training post, which with MMC (modernising medical careers) will mean any doctor in the foundation or specialist training grades. The terms senior house officer (SHO) and specialist registrar (SpR) will be phased out with the introduction of the new run-through training grades. For more information see Chapter 15.

Application for foundation jobs takes place during the Autumn of the final year. The application process has been discussed in Chapter 15. A successful graduate is eligible for provisional registration with the General Medical Council (GMC) which lasts for 12 months. These appointments should be well supervised, but there can still be a great variety in the number of hours worked, intensity of work, training provision and level of senior support. It is therefore worth spending some time researching the potential post, especially if it is in a hospital or area of the country where you have not worked. At a minimum, visit the hospital and talk to staff who are already employed by that trust. The work involved with each post will also vary depending on the speciality. Some may require less in the way of out-of-hours commitment e.g. general practice, psychiatry while during other posts you will be working night shifts and weekends. There could also be great variety in the amount of responsibility and support given. If in doubt about a clinical decision, liase with a more senior member of the team, working up the chain of command.

The first day

The FY1 posts commence on the first Wednesday of August. Each hospital should run an induction course for the new doctors. For FY1 posts, the induction will often be on the day prior to commencing work, so there are at least some junior doctors available for duty on the first Wednesday. The inductions vary between hospitals but will include a variety of lectures and small group work. The topics covered will include hospital orientation, hospital computer systems including log in and passwords, the process for requesting tests, accommodation and pay, car parking and dealing with death and the coroner. There will be a great deal of paperwork that will need to be completed with the most important form being that of your bank details, so you get paid.

Things to organise by your first day (or soon after)
- GMC registration
- Indemnity insurance – this covers you from a legal point in the event of mistakes. Limited cover is provided by the NHS establishment employing

you but it is ESSENTIAL to take out extra cover with an organisation such as the Medical Defence Union or Medical Protection Society
• Pay roll
• Accommodation and car parking
• ID badge and computer access
• Copy of work rota – to enable essential swaps asap
• Hepatitis B immunity
• Criminal Record Bureau certificate.

After induction and sorting out the paperwork, it is time to pick up your bleep/pager, find the wards and your team. Teams of doctors in hospitals are referred to as a firm and traditionally consisted of one to two consultants, a SpR, and some SHOs and JHOs (possibly one or two), with each firm responsible for patients under their care. With the advent of MMC, the firms will consist of F1 and F2 doctors and then trainees at various stages of their specialist training. There may be little in the way of formal induction to the ward – straight in at the deep end! However you should have had a chance to undertake some shadowing experience with your predecessor, so it won't all be new.

17.2 Life as a foundation doctor

As a qualified doctor, the hospital staff will now treat you a little differently. While you are a medical student, it is easy to feel in the way and a spare part, but once qualified your skills will be much in demand. There will be support around, especially during the first few weeks and usually someone more senior from whom advice may be sought. The first few days can be daunting but will no doubt pass quickly. You will wonder where all the knowledge from medical school has gone and why most of it is no longer relevant. The theoretical information has been taught and now it is time to put it into practice – you can only really learn how to become a junior doctor by performing the job itself. This is when you will start wishing you had spent even more of your student days in the hospital. The transition from being a senior medical student to once again being at the bottom of the chain of command can also be difficult, especially for mature students. As an F1 year doctor, you need to take instruction from your senior colleagues and certainly the majority of the job can be mundane, involving a great deal of chasing results and ordering investigations. It is essential to become competent at the basics before progressing, hence the introduction of MMC. It is important to realise that you are an important member of the team. Being a good foundation trainee involves excellent organisation, communication and team working skills. You are not expected to have an exhaustive knowledge and it is imperative to know your own limits and ask for help appropriately. Knowing your patients medical history and management thoroughly, not only impresses your seniors but will also help improve your enjoyment of the job.

Medical jobs

The junior doctors are responsible for the patients under the care of their consultant. The consultant will perform a ward round once or twice a week with the rest of the firm. It is the foundation doctors' responsibility to know who and where the patients are and to be able to tell the other members of the team the reason for admission, the medical history and relevant investigations that have been performed. A management plan will be made for each patient and, following the ward round, all the jobs must be performed. This will involve chasing and ordering tests, and performing practical procedures. If, during the admission, any patients become unwell, then the nurses will contact the doctor via the pager for review. The bleep, although initially a novelty, will soon become hated.

Surgical jobs

The luxury of a 9 am start will not be afforded in surgery. Surgical ward rounds tend to start at 8 am. The ward round is when a senior surgical doctor will do a tour of all the firm's patients at this time; the consultant will usually attend just two or three of these per week. After the ward round, it is again the job of the foundation doctors' to order tests and chase results. During the week there will be sessions called pre-clerking. This is where patients are seen the week before their routine operation and bloods can be taken and other tests performed. At this time it can be checked that the patient is fit enough for the operation and an anaesthetic opinion can be sought if necessary. The rest of the week involves looking after and treating patients who are at pre- and post-operation stage.

Other jobs

As previously mentioned, at least a couple of posts during the foundation programme will be in medical and surgical specialities. As the foundation programme picks up speed, the potential options for jobs are almost endless and in some ways depend on whether certain departments want to develop training for junior doctors in their specialities. The smaller the speciality, the fewer posts available for foundation doctors. Study the application site for the options.

The on call

A hospital must be open, and emergency health care provided, 24 hours a day, and hence, the doctor's working day is not 9–5. To provide this after hours medical care, each day there will be a team of doctors on call (on take) for each speciality. It is their responsibility to admit patients who are referred to the hospital from either casualty or general practitioners. The term on call has been traditionally used because most of the rotas worked in hospital were of the on-call variety. With the changes in working practice, many rotas are no longer on call, but, for ease of describing out-of-hours work, this term will be used in this chapter.

The foundation trainee tends to be the first doctor to see the patient when they arrive at the hospital. This involves taking a history (asking relevant questions), performing examinations and investigations, and attempting to diagnose and treat the patient. After the on-call period, the more senior doctors will perform a post-take ward round where further management plans can be made. If an acutely unwell patient is admitted, then it is sometimes more appropriate to seek senior help early and initiate treatment immediately.

A further responsibility while on call is to look after the patients on the wards, known as ward cover. Out of hours there will only be one or two doctors responsible for the medical care of all the hospital inpatients. Again the jobs will vary from reviewing sick patients to looking up results and performing practical procedures. Depending on the speciality, on call could involve either admitting patients, ward cover or both.

Unfortunately, life as a junior doctor is not quite as glamorous as it is portrayed in many medical dramas; indeed, much of the work can be fairly boring; for example looking up blood results and writing them up in notes. Nevertheless there will be times when you are dealing with very poorly patients who need urgent medical attention, and there is no better feeling than when you have initiated treatment and seen a patient improve. On the downside there will also be times when patients die despite all the intervention that you have attempted. Most of a junior doctor's work is essentially clerking but there will be bursts of fear and adrenaline. Although most of the time, support will be near, there could be occasions when you are the only doctor around and it will be necessary to think and act quickly. It is important to be able to work as a team member and liase and delegate with other staff to perform the necessary tasks. It is easy to say, but it will be essential to keep a cool head, and in most circumstances it will be possible to think first and act later. Roughly translated, take a step back and think about the situation, rather than rushing in and doing something that could be potentially dangerous. And if in doubt, look to one of the experienced nurses for advice – they can be your best friend, or your worst enemy!

Remember that a foundation doctor will often be the initial contact for patients, relatives and other healthcare professionals, so appearance, good communication skills and bedside manner are essential attributes.

Things to consider as a junior doctor

- Be friendly and smile
- Take your breaks and organise holiday leave early
- Be reliable
- Call for help sooner rather than later – your seniors do not like surprises!
- Have interests outside medicine and enjoy your free time
- Never shout at colleagues
- Prepare for the future

Cardiac arrests

It is important as a doctor to keep a cool head and, as mentioned previously, for the majority of scenarios it will be possible to take a step back and consider a management plan. However, one situation where urgent action is required is in the event of a cardiac arrest. This means that a patient's heart has stopped. Each hospital will have a team of doctors who are on call to cover such emergencies – surprisingly these doctors are often fairly junior and most foundation trainees will find themselves involved at some point.

When your shift begins, you will be handed the 'cardiac arrest bleep' from a colleague, who will no doubt tell tales of horror from the previous shift. Unlike your everyday pager, the cardiac arrest bleep lets out a series of ear piercing tones, often followed closely by a voice telling you where the emergency is located. As a newly qualified doctor, you will certainly have a great deal of anxiety related to carrying this bleep and will experience a sudden adrenaline surge when it actually sounds. The idea is to then run to the appropriate ward, although the initial feeling is to walk slowly in the opposite direction, hoping other more senior people will arrive first. We will not discuss actual management of these situations but advise that it is still important to try and keep a cool head, think logically and elect a team leader to help guide the staff. To help with managing these emergencies, most doctors are offered the opportunity to take part in an advanced life support course which will run through real life situations with mannequins – although also a little nerve wracking, these courses can be good fun and of course the patients can always be resuscitated!

Communication skills

One of the most important skills to be gained during your student days (and beyond) is the ability to be a good communicator. Unfortunately, this has not always been reflected in the medical school course. In fact many of the complaints from patients and relatives (and indeed other medical personnel) are probably a direct result of a breakdown in communication. Firstly it is necessary to explain to your patient (and relatives if appropriate) about any information as it becomes available. Medical jargon should be avoided and explanations pitched to the level appropriate to your patient (don't patronise). It is essential that doctors and other medical personnel involved in the care of the patient liase with each other regarding diagnoses, test results, information relayed to patients, etc. Documentation in notes is crucial since, in the age of increasing litigation, this will probably be the only evidence available – it is not guaranteed that a doctor will remember the events a year later (or even the specific patient). Occasionally mistakes may happen and patients and/or relatives will be unhappy with situations. Apologise if necessary and always remember that honesty is the best policy.

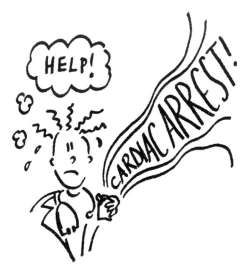

Life as a junior doctor

Accommodation and pay

Accommodation on the hospital site is usually provided for the first year following graduation, although there can be significant variation in the quality. The advantages of living on site is the proximity to work, the social life and the fact that it is provided free of charge. Proximity to work could also be classed as a disadvantage, as could the general quality of the buildings. Many of the regulations were set out as part of the Government's New Deal but, like the hours saga, many hospitals are way behind in their improvements. Traditionally, accommodation for pre-registration doctors has been free because of the extensive hours worked but due to the recent reductions in hours this may not be the case in the future.

After 5 years of poverty, the first wage packet will be a great comfort. The only problem is that the majority of the content will be spent paying off the debts built up over the last few years. If the accommodation is free, then it is a good opportunity to pay off some of the debts during this first year. A supplement to your income will be cremation form fees: when a patient dies a cremation form must be completed and signed by the doctor to permit the cremation to proceed. This is a legal document and, like any other legal document in medicine, a fee is charged. Just don't forget to tell the tax man!

17.3 Specialist training

As doctors progress up the career ladder, their duties can change. With seniority comes increased responsibility and decision making. The advent of reduction in hours and the introduction of modernising medical careers could see junior doctors becoming less experienced. There is also a call for more senior doctors to have a greater 'hands on' contact with patients. For this reason some junior doctors still find frustration with their work when they still have to 'run things by the boss'. No matter what grade, there will still be laborious tasks to complete but in general there will be greater exposure to more complex patients and also more complicated procedures. During specialist training, most doctors will be required to study for postgraduate diplomas. It can be difficult to juggle clinical commitments and family life during this time, so good time management will be essential. It is not uncommon for doctors to take several attempts to get through these exams, which then also adds a financial burden as the cost has to be met personally. In fact this could often be the first time an exam has been failed during a medic's life, which can be hard to accept by some – try not to be disheartened, it often has no reflection on your ability as a clinician.

Three or four years postgraduation is also a time when some doctors decide to change their career path. By this stage they have had a chance to think more carefully about their future career and have had more experience of the different specialities. The change is often due to lifestyle decisions, family commitments, disillusionment with a particular career or difficult career progression due to competition.

17.4 Senior medical appointments

So 5 years of undergraduate medicine and multiple exams, followed by up to 12 years of postgraduate training and further exams, and you have finally made it – an independent practitioner! So surely now it is all about BMWs and ultimate power – who would question such a knowledgeable specialist. The reality is unfortunately different. Although doctors will earn a comfortable wage, few will earn the big bucks without large private practices (with the new consultant contract, private practice will not actually be allowed for the initial years as a senior clinician). There are still large parts of the job that can be routine and there has been an increasing amount of paperwork introduced. Of course a greater proportion of the work will involve managerial aspects, education and dealing with the politics involved in running departments and practices. Another fairly recent change is the necessity for continuing medical education. Medicine is such a rapidly advancing field that it is essential that all doctors show they are keeping up to date. This will involve continuing research and attending various meetings and conferences and may even involve the introduction of further assessments. Hopefully though, a doctor will have chosen their particular speciality due to a keen interest and therefore in general will be enjoying their work.

17.5 Difficult times

In general the majority of doctors enjoy most of their working time. It is common to experience difficult times but these are often transient. There will be times when stress levels are high and this is particularly the case when patients die, especially if unexpected. The responsibility and demands of the job can lead to exhaustion especially with increasing litigation, complaints and patients' expectations. It is important to talk to colleagues and friends and possibly even have a debriefing session following difficult clinical scenarios. If feedback is not forthcoming from senior colleagues, then arrange a time to sit down with the bosses and discuss your progress. It may even be necessary to take some leave or have a break from medicine. It is also essential to keep active interests outside medicine.

17.6 Summary

For many, the first year post graduation is both the best and worst year of their lives. After a gruelling 5 years at medical school, you are finally earning money and hopefully making a difference. The majority of hospitals house the junior doctors in close proximity to each other, which should mean a good social life. For many the glory and the glamour are not as they had imagined and the routine, sometimes boring, jobs are not stimulating. Comments such as 'a monkey could be trained to do my job' are not very encouraging for future doctors. In defence of the hospitals, many have introduced new methods to try and reduce the long hours worked by the doctors and, in doing so, have cut down on some of the more laborious tasks that would not be classed as being educational and so not suitable for a training doctor. Nevertheless a great majority of the work as a junior doctor will be routine, but the skills gained in the first couple of years are essential to a future career in any of the specialities. Like many professions, it is necessary to be an apprentice for some part of your training and, after all, it only lasts a short time.

This chapter has tried to give an honest view of the reality of being a doctor. Remember that the majority of doctors succeed in their chosen speciality and have enjoyable careers. The job of a doctor has great variety and is very reward- ing. Always want the best for your patients and try not to get too demoralised with the government using the NHS as a political tool and the obvious finan- cial implications of this.

PERSONAL VIEW   *Gemma Wilkinson*

There were lots of good things about the idea of starting work: earning money (it's needed after 5 years at medical school!), the thought that at last you might get to do something useful rather than get in the way on the wards and then there was the social life to look forward to, because everyone knows what a great time you have as a junior doctor. So why on the night before I started work did I feel so nervous? I'd spent 5 years training for this moment and I thought that by the time I started I'd know everything, be raring to go, but nothing could have been further from the truth.

My first day passed by in much of a blur. On the first day of any new job you have to sit through the dreaded induction session. Hours of lectures about the 10 different ring tones of a fire alarm and their individual meanings, and how to obtain a car parking permit allowing you to park, at great personal expense, 10 miles away from the hospital. I may have even avoided going to my ward altogether, certainly no real work was done. We all got home and were feeling rather pleased with ourselves. We'd survived the first day and things could only get better. All of us except my flat mate. She had pulled the short straw: on call on the first night. The following morning I checked her bed; it had not been slept in, hardly a good sign. A friend knocked on the door and close on his heels was my housemate looking somewhat dishevelled. She told us how she had been up all night doing these blood tests called APTTs. Every time she thought she had finished, another ward would call her and the same test would need doing. As she spoke she already sounded so knowledgeable, she'd done these

(Continued)

(*Continued*)
tests and checked the results and then altered the patient's treatment. She'd had no sleep and no food, but as she rushed off to try to have a shower before the day started again, I didn't feel sorry for her, only alarmed. My friend and I looked at each other and said simultaneously 'What's an APTT?'

That was how most of my conversations started that first week as I remember, 'What's a . . .?' An APTT is a common blood test, which can help you manage a patient's treatment and, when you've done it once, there's nothing mysterious or difficult about it, but that week a lot seemed mysterious and difficult. One of the things I was most worried about was my first on-call duty. In the day there was always someone around to ask, someone to hold your hand, but on call, at night, alone seemed an entirely different prospect.

I remember vividly my first on call. I was covering the wards. This means that, if there are any jobs to do for the patients on the wards or if a patient becomes unwell, you are the first port of call for the nurses. As 5 pm approaches you start to be bleeped by your colleagues. They might want you to check a blood result that won't be back until later, or to tell you about a patient they are worried about. I got a bleep from one of the SHOs. He asked me to check a patient's blood gases at 6 pm. This is a blood test, but needs to be taken from an artery from the wrist, so is a bit different from a usual blood test. Anyway I had never done one before, but knew in theory what to do. At 5.55 pm I set off to the ward. My palms were sweating and my hands were shaking as I arrived on the ward and went to look for the needle. I'd just got everything ready when a nurse tapped me on the shoulder. 'You don't need to do that anymore,' she said, 'the gentleman has just passed away.' 'Oh thank God for that,' I said. She looked at me rather strangely and walked off. I spent the rest of the night feeling incredibly guilty that I'd been pleased that the man had died, because then I didn't have to do my blood test. Of course I did not mean what I'd said – it was in the heat of the moment in sheer panic.

The first weekend on call meant little sleep for an even longer period of time. At some time in the morning I was bleeped to attend a ward to see an elderly gentleman who was struggling with his breathing. I arrived and indeed he did not look very well at all. I asked a few questions and did a quick examination but felt that I needed to act quickly to help him. I must have looked like a scared rabbit caught in the car head lights. It seemed all that I had learnt during university had disappeared out of my head. I bleeped my SHO frantically; she was busy but would come as soon as possible. In the meantime she gave me various suggestions to try and diagnose the problem. Of course these were all very sensible things that I already knew, but in the heat of the moment I had

(*Continued*)

(*Continued.*)

forgotten. By the time she arrived I had managed to do a blood gas and take a heart tracing. With some nebulisers and oxygen the patient did start to improve. I guess the lesson was that, unless a patient has actually stopped breathing, there is normally some thinking time and it is worth taking a step back and thinking things through logically before panicking.

Starting any job is never easy, but things get better very quickly: you learn fast and there is always someone around to ask for help. As a wise man said, you only have to do your first week once – obvious but true.

Chapter 18 **Career options**

It is unusual for a prospective medical student to know what their ultimate speciality will be. Of those who think they do know, most subsequently change their minds. By the end of medical school the majority of students have a general idea of the broad area of medicine they wish to continue in e.g. general practice, hospital medicine. Graduating from university with a medical degree allows a diverse range of possible career opportunities to suit people with all types of personalities and interests. Unfortunately some medical graduates are not actually aware of all the possibilities available. This may be due to the small size of certain specialities and the lack of coverage during the medical school curriculum. It is essential to be aware of the options and prospects before embarking on postgraduate training and although not intended to be exhaustive, we hope this chapter outlines the majority of choices. With the current changes happening in medical training, there are still areas of uncertainty with regard to length of training and progression. It will be worthwhile reviewing the individual speciality websites (see Table 18.2) for up to date information. The statistical information used in this chapter can be found on the Department of Health's website. For more information we recommend reading the BMA's (British Medical Association) guide to career choice (found on their website) and also *So you want to be a brain surgeon?* (Blackwell Publishing).

18.1 The career ladder

The generic career ladder has been described in Chapter 15. All doctors will enter foundation training for 2 years following university. If successful they will then embark on specialist training in either a run-through grade or via fixed year appointments. The number of years spent during run through will depend on the speciality chosen (approx. 5–8 years). Some doctors will also spend time studying for a higher degree which will mean an extra 2 years for an MD or 3 years for a PhD. Each rung of the ladder will need to be successfully completed in order to progress. This could involve completion of certain exams or assessments and will always involve attainment of the competencies

Table 18.1 The number of doctors working at the different grades 1995 and 2005 in the UK

	1995	2005
GPs	28 869	35 302
Consultants	19 524	31 993
Registrar level	11 466	18 006
SHO level	13 342	21 642
PRHO/F1 level	3 298	4 663
All NHS doctors	*84 459*	*122 345*

set out by each speciality which will be reviewed at an annual RITA (Record of In Training Assessment) meeting. The majority of doctors become GPs with the next 2 largest specialities being medicine and surgery. For this reason there are separate chapters outlining the training in these (Chapters 19–21). Table 18.1 summarises the number of doctors working at different grades in the UK in 2005.

The total figure in the table includes other groups of doctors for example staff grades, associate specialists and dental practitioners. There has been a steady increase in recruitment over the last 10 years, although with the current financial climate in the NHS, it is unlikely this progression will continue, and more worryingly there is actually talk of doctors losing there jobs or retiring doctors not being replaced. As of 2005, 26% of consultants and 55% of PRHOs were female, demonstrating the increased number of female places at medical school but the general lack of femalesenior hospital clinicians.

18.2 The choices

A major advantage to having a medical degree is the large number of possible career options available. Choosing a particular path requires considerable thought as it can have a huge impact on a doctor's eventual professional and personal life. The choice will depend upon an individual's personality and interests. It is necessary for a doctor to decide what they eventually want to get out of the job and the level of responsibility and commitment they wish in the future. It is also essential to think about the career many years down the line as personal aspects will change for example family commitments. Other factors to consider include the amount of patient contact, opportunities for research, flexible working arrangements, ease of taking time out, individual interests, number of postgraduate examinations and level of competition. During university most students will find certain subject areas that they have a greater interest in and also may meet inspirational clinicians during their education. Try to have a broad idea of your speciality towards graduation but avoid a definite decision too early. Currently it is possible to change career paths, but this may become more difficult with run-through training. As well as the large number of medical choices, some graduates decide that being a doctor is not what they envisaged and they leave the profession altogether. Many other professions recognise the qualities that medical graduates possess and offer employment without it being necessary to gain a further degree. A future development could be the increased use of psychometric testing in helping a medical student or doctor choose a career. These tests are becoming more popular as an assessment to determine suitability for gaining a place a medical school.

Choosing a career – things to consider

- Competition for jobs, now and higher up the training ladder
- Amount of patient contact
- Level of responsibility
- Personality
- Possibility for research and teaching
- Opportunities for time out of training
- Opportunities for flexible training
- Out-of-hours commitment, especially at consultant level
- Balance between professional and personal life
- Job satisfaction
- Can you imagine working in this speciality for the rest of your life?

18.3 The options

These can be divided broadly into general practice or medical specialities (community or hospital based), as summarised in Table 18.2. Remember other options such as joining the Armed Forces, being a doctor on board a cruise ship, working in rural areas in other countries, voluntary work in areas of need or working in non-NHS environments e.g. the pharmaceutical industry, medical journalism or medical law. All hospital specialities require at least one postgraduate qualification. The timing of these exams varies between subjects and will certainly change with modernising medical careers. Currently some specialities actually require a postgraduate diploma before entering registrar level training e.g. for haematology, MRCP (Member of the Royal College of Physicians) is required during broad-based medical training and then MRCPath needs to be passed during the haematology specialisation.

Table 18.2 Summary of the specialities available and the postgraduate examinations necessary

Speciality	Generic speciality	Sub-speciality	Useful info	Postgraduate qualification
Allergy	Medicine		www.jchmt.org.uk/allergy	MRCP
Anaesthetics	Anaesthetics		www.rcoa.ac.uk	FRCAnaes
Audiological medicine	Medicine		www.jchmt.org.uk/audio	MRCP or equivalent
Cardiology	Medicine	Stroke medicine	www.jchmt.org.uk/cardio	MRCP
Cardiothoracic surgery	Surgery		www.jchst.org	MRCS
Chemical pathology (clinical biochemistry)	Pathology	Metabolic medicine	www.rcpath.org	MRCPath
Child and adolescent psychiatry	Psychiatry		www.rcpsych.ac.uk	MRCPsych
Clinical cytogenics and molecular genetics	Pathology		www.rcpath.org	MRCPath
Clinical genetics	Medicine		www.jchmt.org.uk/clingen	MRCP
Clinical neurophysiology	Medicine		www.jchmt.org.uk/clinneuro	MRCP
Clinical oncology	Medicine		www.rcr.ac.uk	FRCR
Clinical pharmacology and therapeutics	Medicine	Stroke medicine	www.jchmt.org.uk/clinpharm	MRCP
Clinical radiology	Radiology		www.rcr.ac.uk	FRCR
Dermatology	Medicine		www.jchmt.org.uk/dermat	MRCP
Emergency medicine	Accident & emergency	Paediatric emergency medicine	www.emergencymed.org.uk	MCEM
Endocrinology	Medicine	Diabetology	www.jchmt.org.uk/endocrin	MRCP
Forensic psychiatry	Psychiatry		www.rcpsych.ac.uk	MRCPsych
Gastroenterology	Medicine	Hepatology	www.jchmt.org.uk/gastro	MRCP

(Continued)

Table 18.2 (Continued.)

Speciality	Generic speciality	Sub-speciality	Useful info	Postgraduate qualification
General (internal) medicine	Medicine	Acute, metabolic and stroke medicine	www.jchmt.org.uk/gim	MRCP
General practice	General practice		www.rcgp.org.uk	MRCGP
General psychiatry	Psychiatry	Liaison and substance misuse psychiatry	www.rcpsych.ac.uk	MRCPsych
General surgery	Surgery		www.jchst.org	MRCS
Genitourinary medicine	Medicine		www.jchmt.org.uk/gum	MRCP
Geriatric medicine	Medicine	Stroke medicine	www.jchmt.org.uk/geriat	MRCP
Haematology	Medicine		www.jchmt.org.uk/haem	MRCPath
Histopathology	Pathology	Cytopathology, forensic pathology, neuropathology, paediatric pathology	www.rcpath.org	MRCPath
Immunology	Medicine		www.jchmt.org.uk/immun	MRCP
Infectious diseases	Medicine		www.jchmt.org.uk/infect	MRCP
Intensive care	Anaesthetics		www.rcoa.ac.uk	FRCAnaes
Medical microbiology	Pathology		www.rcpath.org	MRCPath
Medical oncology	Medicine		www.jchmt.org.uk/medonc	MRCP
Medical ophthalmology	Medicine		www.jchmt.org.uk/ophthal	MRCP
Neurology	Medicine	Stroke medicine	www.jchmt.org.uk/neuro	MRCP
Neurosurgery	Surgery		www.jchst.org	MRCS
Nuclear medicine	Medicine		www.jchmt.org.uk/nuclear	MRCP/FRCR
Obstetrics and gynaecology	Obs & Gynae	Gynaecological oncology, maternal and foetal medicine, reproductive medicine, sexual and reproductive health, urogynaecology	www.rcog.org.uk	MRCOG

Occupational medicine	Medicine	www.facoccmed.ac.uk	AFOM
Old age psychiatry	Psychiatry	www.rcpsych.ac.uk	MRCPsych
Ophthalmology	Surgery	www.rcophth.ac.uk	FRCOphth
Oral & maxillofacial surgery	Dentistry/surgery	www.rcseng.ac.uk/dental	MRCS
Otolaryngology (ENT)	Surgery	www.jchst.org	MRCS
Paediatric cardiology	Surgery	www.jchst.org	MRCS
Paediatric surgery	Surgery	www.jchst.org	MRCS
Paediatrics	Paediatrics	www.rcpch.ac.uk	MRCPaeds
	Community child health, neonatal medicine and specialities by organ system		
Palliative medicine	Medicine	www.jchmt.org.uk/palliative	MRCP
Pharmaceutical medicine	Medicine	www.jchmt.org.uk/pharma	MRCP
Plastic surgery	Surgery	www.jchst.org	MRCS
Psychiatry of learning disability	Psychiatry	www.rcpsych.ac.uk	MRCPsych
Psychotherapy	Psychiatry	www.rcpsych.ac.uk	MRCPsych
Public health medicine	Medicine	www.fph.org.uk	MFPH
Rehabilitation medicine	Medicine	www.jchmt.org.uk/rehab	MRCP
Renal medicine	Medicine	www.jchmt.org.uk/renal	MRCP
Respiratory medicine	Medicine	www.jchmt.org.uk/respir	MRCP
Rheumatology	Medicine	www.jchmt.org.uk/rheum	MRCP
Trauma & orthopaedic surgery	Surgery	www.jchst.org	MRCS
Tropical medicine	Medicine	www.jchmt.org.uk/infect	MRCP
Urology	Surgery	www.jchst.org	MRCS

AFOM: Associateship of the Faculty of Occupational Medicine; ENT: Ear, nose and throat; MFPH: Membership of the Faculty of Public Health.

178 The essential guide to becoming a doctor

Table 18.3 Number of doctors working in each speciality as of 2005

Speciality	Consultant grade	Registrar grade	Female consultants
All	31 993	18 006	8353 (26%)
A&E	689	711	151 (22%)
Anaesthetics	4502	2221	1241 (28%)
Clinical oncology	438	281	159 (36%)
Dental	671	345	148 (22%)
General medicine group	7072	4155	1634 (23%)
Obstetrics & gynaecology	1458	1290	432 (30%)
Paediatrics	2033	1617	843 (41%)
Pathology	2398	966	852 (36%)
Public health	927	252	425 (46%)
Psychiatry	3759	1032	1372 (36%)
Radiology	2058	935	620 (30%)
Surgery	5988	4201	476 (8%)

Although not compulsory, most GPs will complete the MRCGP (Member of the Royal College of General Practitioners). Table 18.3 shows the number of doctors working in each speciality as of 2005.

Accident and emergency (A&E) or emergency medicine

As the name suggests doctors in A&E see patients who have a medical emergency or some form of accident. This can range from life threatening conditions including major trauma, to injuries from minor accidents. Some of these patients will have been taken to the department by emergency ambulance but many with more minor problems present themselves. Patients in A&E are triaged (assessed by a nurse to be seen in order of priority) so the more unwell patients are dealt with first. Traditionally there used to be long waiting times in British A&E departments before patients with minor ailments were seen. The introduction of the government's 4 hour maximum wait target has put increased pressure on the workforce and departments may get fined if patients are waiting over this time. Working in A&E can be hectic and has an unpredictable nature as a patient with any problem could attend. Traditionally most A&E consultants were from a surgical background but currently many more trainees are from other backgrounds. There is a lot of opportunity for practical procedures, especially suturing, and as many patients are transferred to other departments, good communication skills with other healthcare professionals is important.

Training: Following the Foundation Programme, the new training in emergency medicine will involve 6 years of specialist training covering all aspects of acute care including anaesthetics, trauma, intensive care and medicine.

During this time it will be necessary to pass the Membership of the College of Emergency Medicine (MCEM).

Skills: Good team working skills, leadership skills, common sense, able to keep a cool head under pressure, communication skills.

Advantages: Fast paced, variety of cases, opportunities to be involved as a doctor at local events, multi-disciplinary, opportunities for flexible and part-time working.

Disadvantages: Little continuity of care because of the high turnover of patients, full shift rotas so more antisocial hours (more weekends and nights than most specialities), stressful.

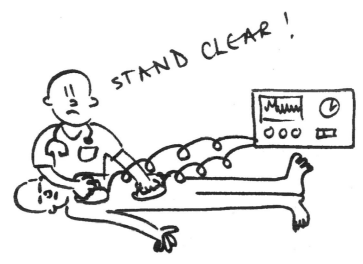

Career paths: A&E

Anaesthetics

Put simply, the anaesthetist's main job is to put patients to sleep ready for a surgical procedure and then wake them up again afterwards. Many operations are now performed under local or regional anaesthesia which has increased the number of procedures possible. There are many other roles for an anaesthetist including an extended role in managing pre- and post-operative care and administering pain relief, acutely in the form of epidurals and also for patients with chronic pain problems. Junior anaesthetists are often involved in helping at cardiac arrests in a hospital and will often be part of the arrest team (a team of doctors and other health professionals called immediately if a patient stops breathing). Like A&E, this is another speciality with little continuity of care unless an anaesthetist has a responsibility for the intensive care unit. Factors such as service provision and shift rotas mean that anaesthetics has good opportunities for flexible training. It is now quite common for a consultant to sub-specialise in one field of anaesthesia, for example cardiothoracic, paediatric or intensive care. It is important to be a team player as it is necessary to deal with hospital staff from all areas, not just the operating theatres. Some of the work can be routine but emergencies can develop quickly, and so the ability to cope with stress is also very essential.

Training: Foundation Programme and then run-through training either in anaesthetics alone or during the early years in combination with other core acute speciality training. Some doctors have traditionally moved into anaesthesia after passing the MRCP. The exams will take place during the run-through training.

Skills: Good team working skills, leadership skills, able to keep a cool head under pressure, communication skills.

Advantages: Opportunities for flexible or part-time working, wide variety of patient care, management of acutely unwell patients, great satisfaction in providing immediate life support to critically unwell patients.

Disadvantages: Minimal continuity of care as patients are handed back to hospital teams after operations or ICU (intensive care unit) admission, long operations sat at the head of the bed, unpredictable nature.

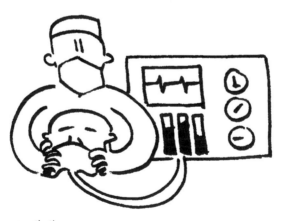

Career paths: anaesthetics

Obstetrics and gynaecology (O&G)

Two specialities for the price of one! Obstetrics involves caring for pregnant women and gynaecology covers diseases of the female genital tract. It is essential to have knowledge of many medical fields, including endocrinology, medicine, neonatology, physiology, sexual problems and also to have the relevant surgical skills. In obstetrics it is necessary to know the physiological changes during pregnancy and then have the necessary skills to perform safe deliveries. From a gynaecological aspect the case load includes sexual problems, urological complaints, menstrual disorders, and gynaecological cancers. Many students enjoy their time on the labour suite dealing with relatively young and healthy patients and also assisting in the delivery of babies. This can be a slightly skewed picture, and it is important not to forget that mothers and babies can run into problems and emotions can run high. It is essential that a doctor in this speciality can deal with stressful situations. Although possible to become a general O&G doctor, many trainees now have a sub-speciality interest especially in the larger tertiary referral centres e.g. gynaecological malignancy or reproductive medicine.

Training: Foundation Programme and then approx 7 years run-through training (2 years Basic Specialist Training (BST), 3 years Intermediate Training (IT) and 2 years Advanced Training (AT)). MRCOG (Member of Royal College of Gynaecologists) Part 1 and set competencies are required to move up to IT and MRCOG Part 2 and further competencies are needed to continue to AT.

Skills: Empathic, ability to work under stressful conditions, communication skills.

Advantages: Relatively young and often healthy patients, wide variety of sub-specialities, emotional rewards, delivering babies.

Disadvantages: Antisocial hours even for consultants, stressful, extremely emotional if things go wrong, litigation, patients expectations.

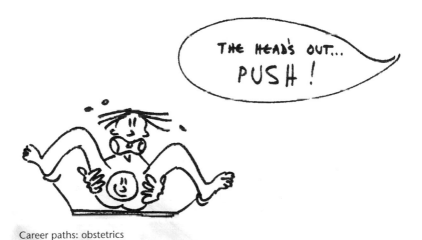

Career paths: obstetrics

Paediatrics

This is the branch of medicine providing care for children. The opportunity for sub-specialisation in paediatrics is more limited than in adult medicine and many of the consultants will act as general paediatric physicians. At large tertiary referral centres there may be doctors with a special interest in certain areas. This branch of training is also followed for neonatology (care of the new-born) and community paediatrics. Many undergraduates enjoy the speciality ('Ah! babies!!'), but in a similar way to O&G, emotions can run high during stressful times and remember most of the patients will come with their parents. It is interesting that it was only fairly recently that Paediatrics became independent of Adult Medicine with the development of their own college – prior to this the postgraduate exam was the same as for adult physicians. Opportunities for flexible training are good as can be seen by the high number of female consultants. Like O&G, this speciality is likely to require more senior input at unsocial hours.

Training: Foundation of 2 years followed by (probably) 6 years run-through training during which time it will be necessary to pass the MRCPaeds.

Skills: Don't have to be a big kid but it probably helps, calm, friendly, able to cope with potential emotional and stressful times.

Advantages: Wide variety of conditions, diagnostically challenging as history not always easy, flexible training, high cure rates.

Disadvantages: Unsocial hours even as senior doctors, emotionally draining.

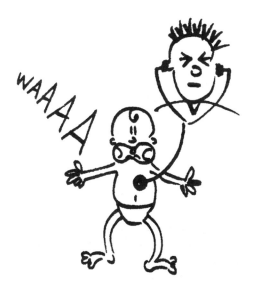

Career paths: paediatrics

Pathology

This is the study of disease processes. The image that comes to mind is the pathologist performing the autopsy (post mortem), and having nothing whatsoever to do with living patients. In reality the subject is much greater and has significant variety. The title pathology is actually an umbrella heading for several subjects that are summarised below. As a generalisation, the majority of the work will involve using specimens from the human body to help clinicians diagnose disease. This may include blood and other bodily fluids and also biopsy specimens. In this way the pathology services will be used by doctors from all fields – communication is thus essential. There is a dedicated exam for these specialities: the MRCPath. There will be opportunities for a small amount of doctors to take posts in these specialities during their F2 year but the majority will enter following the Foundation Programme and embark on run-through training which will last for 5 years. The MRCPath is divided into 2 parts which need to be completed at certain stages in order to continue.

Chemical pathology

This is otherwise known as biochemistry and it involves the running of biochemical laboratories involved in the interpretation of investigation results. Doctors in this speciality also have clinic commitments where they manage and advise other clinicians about various metabolic disorders, for example patients with high cholesterol. It is also common for trainees to complete some research during their training.

Haematology

This speciality used to be laboratory based but now the clinical component predominates. There is a significant inpatient and outpatient workload. Great variety can be seen with the conditions and one appealing factor is the complete management of the patient from the first abnormal blood test, to diagnosis of the disorder, both clinically and by performing tests such as a bone marrow aspirate. The spectrum of disease ranges from abnormalities in the numbers of blood cells in the body, through clotting disorders and genetic problems, to haematological malignancies and blood transfusion conundrums. This speciality requires 2 sets of postgraduate exams to be passed – the MRCP during the first 2 ST (Specialist Training) years (core medical training years – see Chapter 20) and then the MRCPath during later training. Your workload as a consultant will depend on the type of hospital and area but it is possible to sub-specialise in a specific area of haematology, for example bone marrow transplantation (some students find this term a little confusing – it should be noted that this does not require an operation and the transplant is supplied through a drip, in a similar way to a blood transfusion).

Histopathology/cytology

Histopathology involves the study of the function and structure of the tissue from a patient's body; cytology involves the study of the structure and function of cells. The examination of these tissues and cells using a microscope and special staining procedures can help to provide the diagnosis. As well as microscopic techniques, pathologists are also involved with performing autopsy examinations (dissection of a body to determine the cause of death). Research is common and, in the larger teaching hospitals, you can often develop an interest in one particular organ or system.

Microbiology

Here you will be involved in the management of clinical infections both in the hospital and the community. Much of the work will help clinicians in other specialities to isolate and determine micro-organisms and to advise on appropriate treatment with antimicrobials (for example, antibiotics). As well as being concerned about patient infections, part of the workload will involve education about the prevention of the spread of infection. Although it may seem from the outside that much of the time would be spent using a microscope, the work of the microbiologist involves clinical decision making regarding difficult cases on the wards. There tends to be a particularly close relationship with doctors with an interest in infectious diseases. There are several sub-specialities including virology and parasitology.

Ophthalmology

Ophthalmologists are concerned with treating diseases of the eye and visual system, from the contents of the orbit to the brain. Ophthalmology is considered to be somewhat of a hybrid of surgery and medicine – indeed there are many medical conditions that affect different parts of the body, such as disorders of the blood, heart, and even joints, that are first apparent with symptoms related to the eye. The majority of patients are elderly, but usually not very unwell, and some require a long period of care, with many appointments in the outpatients department. Operations are usually short and conducted under local anaesthesia, and the surgery itself is usually very fine surgery, conducted under an operating microscope, or with a laser, to treat diseases affecting the retina (the back of the eye). Ophthalmology, although considered to be a sub-speciality of medicine and surgery, is now becoming further subdivided into the fields of corneal surgery (such as corneal transplantation), surgery of the orbit (for example, orbital tumours), vitreoretinal surgery (treating such things as retinal detachments), paediatric ophthalmology and finally medical ophthalmology involving not surgery but treatment of diseases of the eye such as vascular and inflammatory disorders. The instruments particular to this speciality are the ophthalmoscope to peer into the eye, and the slit lamp which allows visualisation of the lens and the back of the eye.

Training: Trainees will enter Ophthalmic Specialist Training (OST) following their Foundation Programme (some may have spent part of their F2 year in the speciality but this will not be essential). This OST will last between 6 and 7 years and will require a trainee to complete the FRCOphth. The examination will be in two parts, with the first one having to be completed by the end of year 2. Failure to gain this will prevent progression. The second part is likely to be sat towards the end of year 4. As with all the specialities, trainees will have to demonstrate satisfactory progress in obtaining competencies in order to continue in their training.

Advantages: Combination of medicine and surgery, diagnosis often possible on examination alone, few emergencies so out-of-hours commitment less, long term care of patients.

Disadvantages: Highly competitive, a lot of cataract operations.

Psychiatry

This involves studying and diagnosing mental illness as well as behavioural and emotional problems. It is a surprisingly large speciality, incorporating hospital as well as outpatient and community based care. There is an emphasis on multidisciplinary team working; doctors are only a small part of a large team of nurses and social workers and communication skills are essential. Most consultants will have a sub-speciality interest e.g. old age psychiatry, child and adolescents, substance misuse, forensic psychiatry. The postgraduate exam is the MRCPsych which will need to be completed during specialist training. It involves a combination of multiple choice, essay, viva and clinical examinations. Compared to other specialities there tends to be less in the way of practical procedures and life on call can be slightly more civilised.

Training: Foundation Programme followed by up to 6 years run-through specialist training.

Skills: Good at communicating, empathic.

Advantages: Flexible working, light on call, interface with many other branches of medicine, good job opportunities, ability to work in large teams and in various locations.

Disadvantages: Chronic problems with the results of treatment often taking weeks to be seen, patients following through with their suicidal ideas, emotionally draining.

Radiology

Radiology doctors use X-rays and other imaging techniques to assist in disease diagnosis. As well as having an eye for detail required for interpreting these scans, some become interventional radiologists. This involves performing invasive procedures under scanning guidance, traditionally skills performed by physicians or surgeons. With the advance in imaging technology, it is now possible to become a consultant with a particular interest in one area, for example magnetic resonance imaging. Radiologists will investigate other consultant's patients and so communicating and liaising with the other teams is essential. This role is not to be mistaken with that of a radiographer who will actually perform many of the scans while the radiologist has the responsibility of interpreting the pictures. As well as a good knowledge of anatomy, a doctor in this speciality needs a good background in medical, surgical and pathological processes and their treatment. For this reason, although not compulsory, many trainees spend time in these specialities first, often gaining a diploma e.g. MRCS. The actual Royal College of Radiologists diploma is the FRCR (Fellow of the Royal College of Radiologists) and this needs to be achieved to progress through to gain a CCT (Certificate of Completion of Training). Due to a recent shortage of Radiologists there has been a recent collaboration between the department of health and the college called The Radiology Integrated Training Initiative (R-ITI). The new training programme in radiology has yet to be finalised.

Skills: Good communication skills, fine eye for detail, dexterity for interventional procedures.

Advantages: Flexibility, rapidly advancing technology, reasonable on call, expanding, autonomy (in control of your own scanners!), well structured training programme.

Disadvantages: Lack of follow up of patients, can be seen as just a service speciality, extra exams.

Academic medicine

To become a professor or work in an academic university department, you will have to take a slightly different path – it is possible to do this in most hospital and non-hospital specialities including general practice. The training path will be longer because it is essential to study for a higher degree (e.g. PhD). Academics still provide patient care but spend an increased amount of time pursuing research interests and contributing to the education and training of other healthcare professionals. The titles of academics are lecturer (equivalent to registrar) and then senior lecturer, reader and ultimately professor (all senior medical appointments and equivalent to consultant). Most academics will be jointly employed by the NHS and the University. Competition for posts is high and time management skills are essential to be able to balance the clinical commitments with research and teaching time.

Pharmaceutical industry

There are many doctors who decide that instead of treating patients directly, they would rather be involved in developing new drugs. Doctors work within all areas of the pharmaceutical industry – in laboratories with scientists discovering new drugs, running clinical trials where new drugs are tested on volunteers to see if they are safe and effective, with regulatory bodies who check that new drugs have gone through all the necessary tests, and in sales and marketing. The financial resources of the pharmaceutical industry can come as a (not unpleasant) shock after working in the cash-strapped NHS and the work can be exciting and intellectually stimulating. Many doctors miss patient contact; others see this as an advantage.

Most doctors enter the pharmaceutical industry after at least 3 years working as an NHS doctor, and postgraduate exams are becoming increasingly necessary. There are plans to introduce specialist registrar training in pharmaceutical medicine.

The Armed Services

It is possible to work as a doctor in one of the Armed Services. This choice can be made during university days and each medical school will normally hold a careers fair early in the 3rd year. If a medical student decides at this point that they wish to pursue this particular path then the chosen Armed Force will sponsor the student through the clinical years (by covering tuition fees and paying an annual salary). In return you have to continue in employment for up to 6 years following graduation. If you leave before this time then you would be responsible for paying some of the money back. Many of the jobs offered by the Armed Forces will be based in the UK. The opportunities for travel will be easier and graduates could find themselves in countries at war. Spending time in the Armed Forces will not usually affect career progression but there may be some specialities in which it is difficult to obtain the correct exposure. Many of the early jobs will involve general practice-type duties. A further difference is that a few months may be spent doing general training with non-medical colleagues.

Non-medical

Despite 5 years at medical school, some people do decide that medicine is possibly not the vocation for them. Qualifying with a medical degree can open doors to a range of other non-medical jobs. Most doctors make the change some time after their first couple of years – this has given them enough experience to be sure and also allows them to achieve full registration in case of future need. Employers will look seriously at medical graduates because of their proven academic records and also the characteristics and skills they will have. On the downside they may question your dedication and staying power. Most of those leaving the hospital and GP circuit will seek careers not altogether foreign. These will include the pharmaceutical industry, medical journalism, medical law and holistic health opportunities. Outside of medicine altogether, possibilities are endless. Some have moved to the bright lights of the capital city for careers in banking and finance, and one doctor in the Midlands even changed to driving a taxi! The reasons for changing career are usually personal. Pay and hours are poignant issues, but from the outside the grass can always appear greener, so be sure of your decision.

18.4 Summary

Until recently the number of doctors in this country was expanding at a rapid rate in order to cope with the reduction in hours governed by the European Working Time Directive. With the financial crisis in the NHS, the expansion has now been reduced and there is a real chance that doctors could find themselves unemployed. For this reason competition for places will increase and so it is essential to keep ahead of the game with regard to opportunities for improving your curriculum vitae. No other degree allows such variation in a graduate's ultimate job selection but it is essential to think carefully before choosing a particular speciality as it could become more difficult to change the further down the training path a doctor goes.

Chapter 19 **Training as a general practitioner**

Each GP provides 'front line' care for about 2000 patients. They manage up to 90% of episodes of illnesses seen by all doctors, and as well as looking after chronic diseases they play a role in health promotion. Approximately 50% of doctors are GPs, although if you asked most first year medical students whether they wanted to be GPs, the proportion would be much lower. The fact is most people start medical school at the age of 18 years and do not know what area they want to specialise in. This is both normal and sensible because you do not know what the various jobs involve. Some people have a very strong idea about their chosen career, but it is surprising how many of these views will change with time.

Try to keep an open mind for as long as possible, there's no hurry! One point to remember is that at medical school the teaching in the clinical years is predominantly hospital based. You may have a 4 to 6-week placement in general practice with one GP, but otherwise you are taught primarily by hospital physicians and surgeons. It is only natural whilst training to find people whom you admire and with whom you identify. It drives your ambition and influences your choice of career. However you may meet over one hundred hospital doctors compared to only one GP. This is obviously a little biased. Luckily things are changing and many medical schools now run teaching in the pre-clinical years where students visit general practices on a regular basis.

General practice can offer a varied and interesting career with flexibility. Just don't forget it as an option.

19.1 The training requirements

The training for general practice is currently under review and is evolving. To become a GP takes a minimum of 5 years after graduating as a doctor. You will need to do your foundation training for 2 years and then complete 3 further years of specialist training. Currently the training combines a number of 6 months post in various hospital specialities as a Senior House Officer (SHO) (e.g. medicine, obstetrics and gynaecology, paediatrics, accident and emergency) and commonly 12 months as a GP registrar (i.e. a training post within general practice, see later). In the near future this is likely to change to become a selection of 4-month hospital posts (as an ST (Specialist Training) doctor) and 18 months as a GP registrar.

To do this you can join a Vocational Training Scheme (VTS), which is a rotation of jobs specially designed for general practice. You apply for the scheme on a national basis and if successful on selection you are allocated jobs in the different specialities in a particular region. You often have some choice in the jobs you would like to do. You will also be allocated a job in general practice under the supervision of a GP trainer. One of the advantages of joining a VTS is that all your jobs are sorted out for you and you do not have to continually apply for new jobs every few months. This not only saves you hassle, but also gives you stability and allows you to live in one area. Other advantages of being part of a VTS include regular teaching, careers advice, information regarding exams and general support. Currently some doctors opt to arrange their own scheme independently, however it is becoming increasingly difficult to do this and you should seek further advice before considering this option. You may also be able to include some experience gained working abroad if applicable, although you would need to check whether a particular job would be accredited for training by discussing this with the PMETB and local post organisers. All this training can be done part time if you have a valid reason for doing so, such as having children.

Often many people entering general practice will have done more than the minimum requirement of jobs. You may start out training to be a paediatrician for example and later decide that it is not for you. Extra experience is seen as a positive attribute for being a GP. You will have additional specialist skills which can only be of benefit during your training and whilst practising as a GP. It is generally thought to be easier to change from a hospital career to general practice compared to the other way around, although this is still possible. As a general piece of advice, if you are unsure whether to be a GP or a hospital doctor, start with the hospital job and take things from there.

In addition working overseas is also viewed in a positive light by GPs, although this will not influence your application. This is becoming more popular amongst all doctors, but has always been welcomed in general practice.

19.2 The GP registrar

Being a GP registrar is a unique post. You will have to work as a GP registrar for at least 12 months. Depending on the VTS scheme you may do your time in general practice at the end of your hospital jobs or you may sandwich your hospital posts in the middle, e.g. 6 months GP at the start and 6 months at the end.

The post usually involves a short period of introduction into the practice. This includes sitting in with GPs, practice nurses, midwives and going out visiting with the district nurses and health visitors. This gives you the opportunity to get to know the staff and find out exactly what everybody's job involves. You then start to see patients as if you were a GP, but usually with longer appointment times at first. You are under the supervision of a GP trainer. These are GPs with a special interest in teaching and who have worked as a GP for at least 3 years. They will carry on doing their normal work, but you can ask them questions if necessary and they will give you regular teaching.

19.3 The exams

At the moment it is not compulsory to sit the college postgraduate membership exam (MRCGP) to become an independent GP, but there are certain competencies that you have to prove by way of an alternative set of exams and oral examinations (including submission of videotaped evidence of consultations). The current MRCGP will be phased out by August 2008 and so by the time most of you read this, it will be compulsory to take the new Membership of the Royal College of General Practitioners exam (nMRCGP) in order to qualify to work as a GP. This new examination will cover both the old MRCGP and the other competencies. This will bring general practice in line with other areas of medicine. In fact, even though it has been optional up until now, many doctors have chosen to sit the MRCGP – we must be a mad bunch!

19.4 The image

I think it would be fair to say that general practice suffers from an image problem. You must have heard people referring to GPs as doctors wearing sandals and cardigans with leather elbow patches! I believe there are several reasons for this.

Many, but by no means all, hospital doctors develop a bad view of GPs. They feel they see unnecessary referrals into hospital, poor quality referral letters and patients with missed diagnoses. These can all be frustrating whilst working in hospitals, especially when very busy and I certainly remember indulging in some 'GP bashing' myself whilst working as a medical SHO. Now, there are some bad GPs, just as there are some bad hospital doctors, but there are often legitimate reasons for 'missed diagnoses' and 'unnecessary referrals'. The lung cancer in a smoker may be quite obvious by the time he/she presents to hospital with 2-stone weight loss, coughing up blood and a round shadow on the chest X-ray, but may not have been so when the GP saw him/her 3 months ago with 'a bit of a tickly cough'. Equally it can be

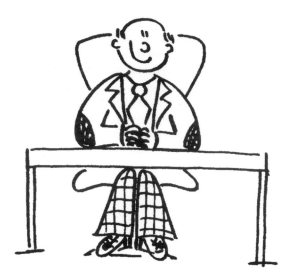

I think it would be fair to say that general practice suffers from an image problem

frustrating that an old lady who fell at home and has broken her wrist has to be admitted to hospital, but if she cannot get to the toilet because she cannot get out of her chair and she has no friends or family to help her then there may be nowhere else for her to go. These things are hardly the fault of GPs, but we are easy to blame.

I believe that the introduction of general practice into many foundation schemes will help to change this. Hopefully now a large number of doctors will gain some first hand experience of working in general practice and the challenges that it raises. This may also help with another common misconception: general practice is boring. A lot of my contemporaries truly seem to believe this. You hear comments such as 'I couldn't cope with seeing all those coughs and colds' or 'don't you get tired of seeing earache?' Boring is one thing that general practice is not. Certainly there are routine parts to it like any hospital speciality, but the truth is you never know what will come through the door next. It might be someone who has just found out she is pregnant, someone whose wife died yesterday, someone with his or her first presentation of a brain tumour or someone having a heart attack. Obviously if you work in hospital and perceive general practice as boring you may also regard those doctors who choose it as inferior. Certainly when I first decided to be a GP I was very careful about whom I told; 'it's a waste' and 'you'll be so bored' were common comments. I do not want to cast all hospital doctors in this light. Many actually admire GPs and go out of their way to be helpful during hospital SHO training posts and later in teaching GPs. Also I do not believe general practice is for everyone (see later), but the point I am making is that general practice often gets bad press in hospitals, and as that is where you spend a great deal of time as a student and junior doctor, some of it no doubt rubs off.

Finally, there has been a lot of coverage in the media recently about low morale in general practice and the lack of GPs. In fact there is usually some medical story in the news each week and this applies equally to hospital medicine, bed shortages, waiting lists and so on. It is important not to become disillusioned and form your own opinions. However, there are other more subtle media influences. On an evening spent at home, if you had a choice would you rather watch 'ER' or 'Doctors'? Not a tricky decision really! Give me the excitement and good looks of those glossy hospital dramas any day. I am not even going to try to pretend that being a GP is as exciting as an episode of ER, thank goodness, but then most A&E jobs are not either. The general public do not think that general practice is as sexy as being a brain surgeon, but you probably realise that.

19.5 Working as a GP

Being a GP is about being a generalist as opposed to a specialist. This may seem obvious but is an important point. A colleague once described general practice as 'specialising in being a generalist'. You are expected to know a little bit about a lot, rather than a lot about a little. This certainly does not appeal to everyone. You will never be a complete authority on a subject. In fact you will end up with a very good knowledge of some of the common general practice problems, but you need to realise your limitations and be prepared to refer on to a specialist if necessary. Increasingly GPs are being encouraged to develop areas of special interest, but you would still be expected to continue with your usual surgeries in addition. With a special interest it is possible to spend some sessions working in the local hospitals under the guidance of a Consultant, for example in A&E.

There are other important aspects about general practice that differ from working in hospitals. As a GP you are self-employed rather than being employed by a hospital. This means that you have more influence over your working conditions, hours and pay. It also means more involvement in managerial and financial skills. In the current political climate, general practice, along with the rest of the NHS, is constantly evolving. In the recent past the way in which GPs are paid has been reformed by a new contract that encourages GPs to meet targets called Quality Outcome Framework (QuOF) points. GPs are currently joining together in groups which will be able to buy in services from hospitals in a scheme called Practice Based Commissioning. There are constantly new challenges to face in the structure and organisation of general practice. This aspect of general practice appeals to some and can have its advantages in the sense of autonomy, but importantly there are an increasing number of jobs that do not require you to become as involved in these aspects if they do not appeal to you.

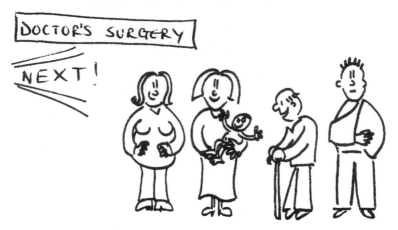

General practice can offer a varied and interesting career

General practices vary enormously and there is no such thing as a typical practice. You can work alone as a single-handed GP or in a large practice with many other partners. You can choose to work in the inner city or in a very rural area. As GPs are self-employed, it means that they can opt to do things in many different ways. This refers more to the organisation of the practice than the medical decisions. For example there are some GP practices around the country where GPs help run small, so-called Community Hospitals. Here they can supervise the care of their own patients in hospital, help run Minor Injuries Units (like a scaled down A+E) and even help out on the maternity wards or other specialist areas. They can have direct access to X-ray facilities and sometimes do their own minor operations.

Thus one of the main advantages of general practice is the flexibility. This can often appeal to women with a view to having children, but may also appeal if you have other interests both medical and non-medical. As a full time GP you will usually work eight or nine sessions per week (a session is a morning or afternoon surgery plus paperwork), which means one or two half days off per week. It is common to find jobs that are three-quarter time, usually six to seven sessions per week or part time, four to five sessions per week. Most practices will do their own on call during the day. In the evenings and the weekends most practices will now use a cooperative or deputising service. Essentially large numbers of practices join together to provide an on-call service. You may be required to do the on call, but this usually only works out at around two to three sessions per month. Basically general practice often appeals to people who want a life outside of medicine or increased variety in their work. This is obviously possible with a career in a hospital speciality, but it is usually harder. However, be under no illusion, being a GP is hard work and is not an easy option, but general practice is often described as a lifestyle choice.

Finally it is important to consider the other aspects involved in general practice. Communication skills are very important. You need to work as part of a team with other health professionals, e.g. other GPs, practice nurses and health visitors, and remember that some of them will be your employees. All doctors need to be able to communicate effectively with patients, but especially in general practice where you will look after your patients for many years. This may not always be an advantage if the patient is difficult, but mostly it offers a unique opportunity for you to build relationships with patients and their families. You also have the opportunity to see patients in their own environment, which is very different to talking to someone in a hospital bed. It allows you develop understanding of how illness can have an effect on a person's daily life, including home, work and relationships.

19.6 Summary

If you had asked me at the start of medical school whether I wanted to be a GP I would have said no. If you were to ask me whether I am happy with my career choice now I would say yes. General practice is challenging, flexible and fun and I can see myself doing it for the rest of my career. Don't rule it out.

PERSONAL VIEW   *James Hopkinson*

I trained at Nottingham Medical School and had a fantastic time as a student. I knew exactly what my career path was going to be; I was going to be an orthopaedic surgeon, a trauma specialist. I was particularly dismissive of general practice – I didn't want to be a 'second rate' doctor!

Things changed when my house jobs started, and I realised how little time would be spent doing 'exciting' trauma cases, and how much time would be spent doing 'boring' ward rounds and paperwork. I also realised that when the trauma usually happened I would prefer to be asleep! With some trepidation I began exploring other possibilities. I spent some time with GPs and saw that they were in control of what they did, and when they did it. I saw the opportunities to get involved in areas of medicine that interested them, as opposed to the hospital doctors who appeared to have little freedom in their working practices.

I joined the Nottingham VTS straight from house jobs and never looked back. The general practice training was split into two 6 months posts at the beginning

(Continued)

(Continued.)
and the end of my 3 years rotation. In between consisted of 6 months each of Psychiatry, General Medicine, Obstetrics and Gynaecology and Paediatrics. The MRCGP exam followed my final 6 months and then I decided to take advantage of the flexibility general practice allows, and did a 6-month post in sports and exercise medicine – a new and unique post. This was funded by the postgraduate dean as part of an on-going programme to create GPs with special interests (GPSIs). I gained my diploma in sports medicine, and decided that I wanted to continue to work within Sports Medicine. Almost concurrently a partnership in a local village became available. I was hesitant to begin with as there are so many opportunities to locum which carry no long term commitment. The practice was very well set up, was forward thinking and most of all I liked the people there. I subsequently applied and was offered the job. During discussion with the other partners I emphasised my desire to continue to work within sports medicine, and they were all supportive and flexible.

My initial contract was for 6 months. I found I very much enjoyed the working environment, but I had a steep learning curve ahead of me. Suddenly I had more responsibilities than just the medical care of my patients. I was now self-employed, running my own business. The practice employs 35 staff – people management is not part of medical training! Fortunately the other partners were very helpful during my settling in period, and made time to help me out. I also found the paperwork mountain that I had been told about but never really believed. It is true when you become a partner the flood gates open!

As the practice owned its own buildings this meant 'buying' into the practice. This involved taking out a mortgage that was bigger than my house mortgage, to 'buy' the preceding partner out. Fortunately, the PCT (Primary Care Trust) pays rent on the premises, which at present interest rates more than covers the cost of the mortgage. This will hopefully create a nice tax-free lump sum when I retire, and the next person buys in.

Within 6 months I was approached by a professional Olympic team that trains locally asking if I would be interested in looking after them medically. I was obviously very interested, but a little scared as I had never looked after an amateur side! I agreed to do it jointly with a well established sports doctor in the area, whilst I gained more experience. Since then I have travelled with several British teams around the world. I have been Medical Officer to the World University Games in Korea and Turkey, and I was also involved in the Winter Olympics in Turin. General Practice allows me the flexibility to earn a good salary whilst pursuing my special interest.

I love my job, and I would not change it for the world.

Chapter 20   **Training in the medical field (becoming a physician)**

To talk about a career in a medical speciality, it is helpful to first define the term general medicine. It can certainly cause some confusion because at university the course is called medicine, but a career in a medical speciality is different. General medicine is a term that has been used historically. It can also be referred to as internal medicine and involves the diagnosis and treatment of diseases of the internal organs. In simple terms it could be thought of as all the specialities, excluding surgery, general practice, anaesthetics, radiology and laboratory sciences. Traditionally this definition was close to the truth. However, in the modern age there has been diversion of many specialities away from general medicine, a good example being paediatrics. The subspecialisation has come about as technology and medicine become more complex and so a consultant needs to be very knowledgeable in one particular area.

General medicine still exists and will continue to do so, although in time may become a speciality in its own right. Each day a hospital is 'on take' for patients who need to be admitted from A&E (accident and emergency) and GPs. These patients have unselected problems and hence general medical complaints.

The training in many of the specialities within medicine will lead to dual accreditation. Roughly translated, this means a consultant physician is a specialist in one area but also takes part in the unselected general medical admission process. Not all subspecialities in medicine have general medical commitments, but this will depend on the individual hospital.

20.1 The hospital structure

The medical department in a hospital is divided into specialities which in turn are divided into medical firms. These consist of a consultant, specialist registrar (SpR), senior house officer (SHO) and foundation doctors (this will change with modernising medical careers but a firm will still consist of a number of junior and senior doctors, headed by a consultant). Not all firms will have the same number at each grade. The majority of the work for the foundation and SHO doctors is to look after the general day-to-day activities on the ward. This will include a daily review of each patient and organising and chasing the results of tests. The registrar and consultant will have more clinic and procedure commitments depending on the speciality.

Common medical specialities (see Chapter 18 for the complete list)

Acute medicine
Cardiology*
Clinical oncology*
Clinical pharmacology*
Dermatology*
Endocrinology
Gastroenterology
Genitourinary medicine*
Haematology*
Health care of the elderly
Infectious diseases
Medical oncology*
Nephrology*
Neurology*
Palliative medicine*
Rehabilitation*
Respiratory medicine
Rheumatology*

*Not always involved in general medicine

20.2 General medicine

Each day there will be a team of doctors allocated to admitting patients. This means that all the new patients referred to the hospital with medical conditions will come under the care of this consultant. Patients can be referred by the GP or casualty, or be admitted following a 999 emergency ambulance call. These patients tend to be seen initially by the junior doctors, who will perform a medical history (ask some relevant questions) and an appropriate examination, and commence treatment as required. Following the history and examination, it is usual to determine a differential diagnosis, that is, several possible explanations for the patient's symptoms. The patients will be reviewed by senior colleagues on a post-take ward round. Following review on this central admissions ward, the patients can then be moved to other wards depending on their medical needs and also their diagnosis, or discharged home if appropriate. Other information regarding on call can be found in Chapters 15–17.

Examples of general medical conditions

Heart attack
Angina
Asthma
Chronic bronchitis
Stroke
Infections
Blood clots
Diabetes
Bowel problems
Confusion

20.3 Foundation Years

Several posts during the foundation programme will be in medical specialities. The majority of a trainee's time will be spent looking after the patients on the ward. Each patient needs to be seen daily, with the senior doctors doing 2 or 3 rounds a week. Your role is important as you have the most contact with the patients, relatives and other health care professionals. A good foundation doctor will have excellent knowledge of their patients including up to date information of the medical problems, results of tests, investigations pending and their social history. It is important to keep good medical records and know when to ask for advice and assistance. When 'on call', it may be necessary to leave the team ward and spend the day or night on the admissions ward. There will be other members of the team to cover the consultant's patients on these occasions. During the foundation programme it is necessary to show adequate completion of the competencies expected as outlined in the training portfolio. Each doctor will be allocated an Educational Supervisor who will organise meetings throughout the year to check on progress. Many of the patients will require practical procedures to be carried out (see list below). These vary in complexity and as a doctor progresses up the training ladder, they should get experience starting with the simple ones first.

20.4 Specialist training (Basic Medical Training, i.e. ST1 and ST2)

The training grades SHO and SpR are to be replaced with specialist training (ST). These posts are being introduced from August 2007. Chapter 15 outlines the new generic training ladder (Figure 15.2). Following the foundation 2 years a doctor interested in pursuing a career in a physician speciality will need to apply for run-through training. The first 2 years of this will be known as Basic Medical Training (BMT), and following successful completion of this a trainee can continue to Higher Speciality Training (HST). There are 3 BMT programmes that a successful foundation doctor can apply for in order to continue to become a physician: 1. Core Medical Training (CMT), 2. Basic Neuroscience Training (BNT) and Acute Care Common Stem (ACCS). The majority of trainees will enter the CMT pathway. BNT will be divided into medical and surgical stems and those completing the medical BNT will go on to pursue HST in neurology related specialities. ACCS is a stem shared with anaesthetics and emergency medicine and so a trainee could follow one of these paths as an alternative or continue HST in medicine. Like the foundation programme, each component of the training will require adequate demonstration of competencies.

Each of the years will be divided into various 4–6 month placements. During CMT a trainee will rotate through different medical specialities in order to increase knowledge and experience.

During the first 2 ST years, a trainee physician will still spend a large part of their time looking after the ward patients. As seniority develops other opportunities will arise, for example spending time seeing patients in the outpatient department and spending time performing specialist procedures, for example, a training respiratory physician will spend time developing bronchoscopy skills (camera looking into the lungs). Communication remains as ever, an essential part of the job with patients and relatives requiring up to date knowledge of their conditions, and also liasing with other healthcare professionals and specialists when organising investigations. To continue in medical training part of the competencies will be to pass the physician postgraduate examination – the diploma of the Royal College of Physicians (MRCP). Obtaining the MRCP (UK) Diploma does not mean you have gained specialist status but this qualification is required for entry to higher ST. The first part will need to be completed during ST1 and 2 i.e. during CMT.

Practical procedures in general medicine

- *Phlebotomy*: taking blood samples
- *Insertion of cannulae*: small tube inserted into a vein to allow the administration of drugs and fluids

- *Arterial blood gases*: puncturing the radial artery to obtain a blood sample to measure the level of oxygen
- *Bladder catheterisation*: insertion of a tube into the bladder to allow drainage of urine
- *Central (venous) line*: insertion of a tube into a large vein, for example, jugular vein, for administration of fluids
- *Lumbar puncture*: small needle used to obtain specimens of cerebrospinal fluid from the spinal cord
- *Needle aspiration*: needle inserted into body cavity to obtain specimen of fluid
- *Drain insertion*: tube inserted into body cavity to drain fluid

20.5 Specialist training (Higher Specialist training)

After completion of CMT or equivalent, a doctor continues through run-through training into HST. During the early part of this it will be necessary for a trainee to complete the rest of the MRCP. The initial part of ST will be broad-based training and as a doctor progresses, the work will become more limited to the actual chosen speciality. As a more senior doctor, i.e. the equivalent of the current SpR grade, your seniority should in general reflect your clinical responsibilities. As well as outpatient and specialist procedure experience, you will be required to see patients with speciality problems under different hospital teams and advise on their management e.g. surgical patients who have developed a medical problem. You will also be responsible for reviewing patients who become unwell or those that your juniors are concerned about. Other aspects of your work will include more managerial roles and taking part in audit, research and teaching. During this time it will also be possible (and in some specialities compulsory) to undertake a period of formal research e.g. PhD. This will mean 2–3 years outside clinical medicine and on calls, which could improve quality of life but can lead to a big reduction in pay (see Chapter 12 for more information about research). As already mentioned not all medical specialities are involved in general medicine and some actually require further examinations to be taken during HST e.g. oncology and haematology. One other point to mention is that although the MRCP has been taken and the medical rotation completed, some doctors do not remain in the medical field and transfer to other specialities such as general practice, radiology or casualty, where the MRCP is a useful but not an essential qualification.

During HST a doctor should gain the clinical specialist knowledge required to become a hospital consultant. It is also necessary to take an interest in audit, research and managerial aspects. Providing the training has been satisfactory, with completion of the assessments and core competencies as recorded in the training portfolios, the end of the programme leads to a Certificate of Completion of Training (CCT – previously known as CCST (Certificate of Completion of Specialist Training)). This means a doctor has their name on the specialist register and can be an independent practitioner. This qualification is recognised throughout Europe.

20.6 Membership of the Royal College of Physicians Diploma

This postgraduate exam has undergone major changes over the last 5 years. It is divided into 2 parts with 3 distinct components (Part 1 written, Part 2 written and Part 2 clinical). Part 1 is divided into 2 papers with 100 questions each. These are in the 'best of five' format and will test knowledge of common disorders in general medicine and clinical sciences. Recent changes mean that the exam is criterion-referenced and negative marking has been abolished. Criterion referencing means an external assessment is made and a pass mark set rather than the old system of norm-referencing where a certain percentage of candidates were allowed to pass. The Part 2 written exam consists of 3 papers of around 100 questions. The format is a combination of 'best of five' and 'n from many' (choose several answers from a list). The questions will involve clinical scenarios and test a candidate's knowledge of diagnosis, investigation, management and prognosis. In this way the Part 2 written tends to be more relevant to the daily work of a trainee. The Part 2 clinical exam is called PACES (Practical Assessment of Clinical Examination Skills) and consists of 5 stations. This type of examination format is similar to the OSCE (Objective Structured Clinical Examination) that most medical schools now use for examining students. Each of the following systems is tested from a clinical perspective – cardiovascular, respiratory, abdominal, nervous and musculoskeletal (incl. eyes, skin and endocrine). To emphasise the importance of communication skills, 2 stations test this modality.

These exams require a significant amount of studying which can prove difficult during a busy clinical job. Doctors are entitled to study leave and most hospitals provide a protected half-day of teaching each week for their trainees. The other downside to having to sit the exam is the cost. There may be some money available for trainees to attend study courses but most of the examination fees have to be met personally. The total cost for the MRCP in 2007 is over £1000 and that is if you are successful in passing all parts first time.

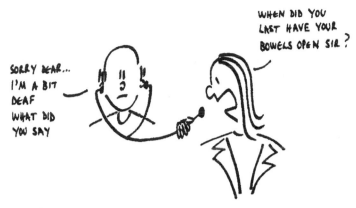

Training in the medical field

20.7 The consultant

After HST it is possible to apply for a hospital consultant post in your chosen speciality. At each step during your training there will be fewer jobs available and hence more competition. To ensure a top teaching hospital job, you often need a further qualification in the form of an MD or PhD. The work of consultants will involve more management and administration than that of their juniors. In total it could take up to 15 years from graduation before taking up a consultant post. Although, once a consultant, you have reached the top of the career ladder, it is still essential that you remain up to date. The days of doctors becoming consultants and possibly never reading another book are over. Continuing medical education (CME) will ensure that consultants keep up to date with the latest treatments. In order to continue practising medicine, you must collect a certain amount of CME points each year. These can be gained from various sources, but usually by attending educational seminars and courses. Most trainees find the transition to being a consultant stressful as the responsibility of the patient now lies with the most senior person i.e. you. Many also find the amount of paperwork associated with being a consultant much greater than they could imagine. In this litigious society other stressful times can involve being called to a coroner's court. Another major role is that of training and teaching medical students, junior doctors and other health care professionals. On the plus side, you are now a specialist in your own right and this will in general mean working less antisocial hours (depending on your speciality) and it is certainly possible to be invited as a guest speaker to various conferences both locally and internationally. Once an independent practitioner it is also possible to set up a private practice. The time and opportunity for this will depend a great deal on personal preference and speciality.

PERSONAL VIEW *John Macfarlane*

Few careers offer such diverse opportunities in life as medicine, including that of a consultant physician. What is a physician? Broadly the term applies to specialists who undertake acute general medicine, managing adults admitted to hospital as medical emergencies with a wide range of acute illnesses (being on take), as well as having particular training and expertise in specialities such as respiratory medicine, gastroenterology, diabetes and endocrinology, healthcare of the elderly and infectious diseases amongst others. Other specialists, such as neurologists and dermatologists (and some cardiologists and nephrologists), are more narrowly based and work only within their speciality, and avoid the thrills and spills of acute medicine.

I became a consultant physician with an interest in respiratory medicine at the age of 33 years, following an enjoyable and interesting training. After obtaining my undergraduate degree, I stayed on at Oxford to do my clinical training and benefited greatly from expert teaching in small groups, and a diverse and busy workload. House jobs followed at the Radcliffe Infirmary, first with the inspirational Paul Beeson, Nuffield Professor of Medicine, and then with two superb, old school general surgeons. By the end of my surgical training, I had become reasonably competent in surgery as well as sorting out the general medicine within the firm. I gained experience and practice in performing emergency appendicectomies (removal of the appendix) (apart from the time I tried to mobilise the common iliac vessels, thinking they were a retroperitoneal appendix (at the back of the abdominal cavity)), hernia repairs and sewing up. I ran my own busy minor operations (ops) clinics weekly, but still remember the first one. 'Don't worry', I was told, 'Your first minor ops clinic is fairly light, with only two temporal artery biopsies and three scalp sebaceous cysts.' 'Where on earth is the temporal artery?' I thought. The scalp has a very rich blood supply, as I learned to my cost.

I had wanted to be a physician for some while and had always been attracted to both chest diseases and infection problems. Although I enjoyed surgery, the thought of having to deal with ghastly postoperative complications put me off, and my sole 2-week exposure to general practice in winter in the north of Scotland had strengthened my attraction to mountains rather than a career in primary care. Brief enthusiasms for radiology and ophthalmology were dampened by my memory of struggling with physics at school. Why infection? I had found microbiology (*Pathology and Bacteriology*) interesting as a medical student and already thought I would work abroad. As for chest diseases, they were common and my teachers enthusiastic. I always gravitated towards chest

(Continued)

(Continued)

patients on the wards, but two scenes stick in my mind – doing my own Gram stains and white blood cell counts as a houseman at the Radcliffe Infirmary in the middle of the night on patients with chest infections, enabling me to take an independent decision about best treatment, and the take night when we admitted a bad case of lobar pneumonia. The senior registrar (now a well known professor in the USA) took some blood, inoculated it into a laboratory mouse and the next morning recovered pneumococci from it. The patient survived his pneumococcal pneumonia with the help of penicillin and I had my first taste of clinical research.

Even in those days the route to medicine was via a good SHO medical rotation and passing the dreaded membership – MRCP. I was fortunate in getting the 1-year SHO rotation in Oxford, which was excellent, followed by a most enjoyable 9-month post at the Brompton Hospital, London. This convinced me that respiratory medicine was for me. I still remember the thrill of passing MRCP and those heady post-membership weeks on the ward as a bumptious, and no doubt irritating, post-MRCP know it all SHO. (In truth, it is probably the pinnacle of your medical knowledge, before the descent!)

We had always wanted to spend time abroad, and, after investigating Papua New Guinea, East Africa, Australia and the Antarctic, I obtained a 2-year registrar (and subsequently senior registrar) post at Ahmadu Bello University Teaching Hospital in Zaria in the Muslim north of Nigeria. Both medicine and life were exciting and challenging, particularly with a wife and small baby. The MRC unit there, run by Brian Greenwood and Hilton Whittle, and the excellent clinical staff (several with links to Oxford) under the legendary Professor Eldryd Parry, led to high-quality medical teaching (I was able to have the time recognised for training once I returned to the UK – an important issue if you go abroad), patient care and a proper introduction to clinical research. I gained a vast amount of clinical experience and learned the crucial skill of spotting the really sick patient. I also gained specialist skills, running the 40 bed TB hospital and the asthma clinic, learnt a lot about tropical medicine, including personal encounters with falciparum malaria and paratyphoid (you could tell if you were quite ill as the resident hospital roof vulture population would become interested in you), and became closely involved in really exciting clinical research into epidemic meningitis (involving over 1200 inpatients), pneumonia and asthma, resulting in nine clinical research papers.

We had accepted that going abroad might set back my career somewhat, as it was not a common thing to do at that time (apart from trips to North America), but I had kept in touch with my consultants in Oxford (it is important and polite to keep in touch with your mentors and referees) and was

(Continued)

(*Continued*)

fortunate in being offered an 18-month locum senior registrar post to return to in Oxford. This was an excellent introduction back into British hospital medicine and I was allowed to rotate from general medicine and cardiology through intensive care unit (ITU) training followed by respiratory medicine. I learnt flexible bronchoscopies (camera used to look into the lungs) on patients sitting in an old armchair in the main chest ward – two anxious people joined by a black umbilical tube.

My next aim was to obtain a substantive senior registrar training post and I ended up in Nottingham – the interview being the day before the one in Aberdeen. This was a busy clinical job with excellent training and allowed me to indulge my interest in respiratory infection. Nottingham had developed a reputation for work into the recently discovered Legionnaires' disease and I was able to continue and expand this work into all aspects of community-acquired pneumonia – an example of exploiting the inevitable. During my 3 years as an SR, I set up and analysed research studies and wrote up my DM (doctorate in medicine) thesis, without any time away from busy clinical work – not to be recommended without rigorous time management and a supportive wife and family. However, walking alone down the red carpet in the Oxford Sheldonian in flowing robes to receive my DM, made all the concentrated effort seem worthwhile to us.

I had not really thought where we should aim to end up for a consultant post – jobs were tight then – but one of the two chest physicians at Nottingham retired early and I was fortunate in being appointed to replace him starting on April Fools Day in 1982.

Nearly 25 years later I am still a physician in general and respiratory medicine, and have had a full, varied and active career. When I started as a consultant, my clinical commitments were much greater than now (there were only two chest physicians for the whole of Nottingham and Newark – today there are at least 14! – and I had numerous clinics, ward rounds and bronchoscopy sessions, and referrals to be seen in other hospitals, sometimes with a bronchoscope and light source in the car boot), but actually life seems much busier now, with the many extra roles a consultant physician is asked to take on. This is the variety and spice of the job, but it can also be wearing and stressful even with careful planning and time management. It is a juggling act of inpatient and outpatient work, seeing referrals, talking to relatives, attending multidisciplinary meetings with other specialists and professionals, teaching undergraduates and postgraduates, reviewing, researching and lecturing, mentoring and appraising trainees, attending management meetings locally, nationally and abroad,

(*Continued*)

(Continued.)

whilst trying to keep up to date professionally, and balancing all this with home, social life and personal time. More recently I also changed my job pattern quite considerably in a number of ways. I became an acute physician for part of the week, spending all day on the acute ward and helping to set up our new acute medical admissions service. 'Hands on' management of acute emergencies certainly refreshes one's skills and knowledge fairly quickly and allows close contact with other health professionals in the team and closer supervision and training of trainees. I was appointed to a personal chair by the University of Nottingham, so my SHOs now call me 'Prof'! I have also become chairman of our specialist society – the British Thoracic Society – which represents over 2600 health care professionals providing respiratory care in the UK and abroad. It is a privilege representing such dedicated colleagues and fun working hard to improve standards and care of patients with lung diseases and lobbying politicians about reducing the burden of lung disease. So still after many years – no day is the same – what more can one ask from a job! But one word of warning! Time will tell whether the new consultant contract and increasingly rigid way of working will make the consultant role more inflexible, and less sustainable by removing some of the variety and energy that enhances the job so much, to the detriment of the consultant and his patients.

- Would I do it again? Yes, certainly – what else could or would I have done?!
- What advice would I give to school leavers thinking of becoming a physician? Be organised and plan ahead, so that, as a doctor, you can do the things you want to do as well as those you have to do.
- Exploit the inevitable – something good can be extracted from every situation.
- Become an expert in something that particularly interests you and stick to it (in my case it was respiratory infections and pneumonia). Experts will always be in demand and it can lead you down many exciting paths such as research, publications, lecturing and advising at home and abroad.
- Finally, when you see your twentieth patient on a post-take round, and you are tired after a full day's work, remember that, although it is a routine encounter for you, it will be an unique and vitally important event for your patient and their family – in their eyes, you are their consultant.

Chapter 21 **Training in the surgical field**

21.1 Introduction to surgery

The dictionary definition of surgery is the 'branch of medicine that treats diseases, injuries, and deformities by manual or operative methods' – that is, using physical intervention as a cure. Surgery can be a very satisfying profession, with a mixture of analytical and manual skills. There can be disadvantages; mainly long hours and commitments that often interfere with your personal life, but all the effort can be worthwhile; as most surgeons will tell you, there is no speciality like surgery, where you can have fun as well as get the chance to perform life-saving and life-improving operations.

21.2 History of surgery

Surgery has been performed since prehistoric times, when sharpened flints and other sharp-edged devices were used to perform such surgical operations as circumcision. The early Greeks and Romans practised surgery with great skill and with such cleanliness that infection of surgical and other wounds was relatively uncommon. During the Middle Ages surgical practice fell into the hands of the unskilled and uneducated. The barber-surgeon, who performed the usual functions of a barber as well as surgical operations, became a common figure, especially in Britain and France. It was not until the 18th century that surgery began to reach a professional level. With the introduction of antiseptic methods, surgery entered its modern phase. Louis Pasteur established the fact that microbes are responsible for infection and disease, and Joseph Lister was the first to discover the principles of antisepsis (the prevention of the spread of infection), prior to which about 80% of surgical patients contracted gangrene. In the 19th century anaesthesia was developed and radically changed surgical practice. In the 20th century, the development of surgical instruments revolutionised the practice, and the introduction of modern imaging techniques and technology, such as heart–lung bypass machines, have made the impossible possible, for example, heart transplantation and tumour excision.

21.3 The career

As with any career, you should think about what you are good at and what you are looking for in your future job. The general attributes of a good surgeon are:
- Making decisions – can you think on your feet and learn from mistakes?
- Life-long learning – would you like to have a career where you need to constantly update your knowledge?
- Building up trust – could you explain things clearly to patients and other doctors in your team?
- Manual dexterity and spatial awareness.

The first three are attributes for doctors in most specialities, but one of the big differences in surgery is the addition of the fourth. If you prefer working alone, hate learning new things, and crack under pressure, surgery may not be for you. However, surgery can be an extremely enjoyable, intellectually demanding and satisfying career.

Surgeons have traditionally been stereotyped as having certain personalities. One opinion is that they should be male, athletic, possessed of a vocabulary of single syllables, have the endurance of a marathon runner, and maintain a political, social and sexual orientation somewhere to the right of Attila the Hun. Is this stereotype fair? Some surgeons may fit the bill, but in general this description is unfair. It is hoped that the methods and manner of characters such as Sir Lancelot from the film *Doctor in the House* are disappearing. The other main fault with the above description can be seen if the number of women now entering surgery is taken into account.

Other changes have come about with the introduction of the Patients' Charter. Surgeons are no longer considered as god-like people who can do only good. It is necessary for them to communicate well and explain why a patient needs the operation they are offering. With the advent of the Internet, patients are much more knowledgeable. Although a considerable amount of time will be spent in the operating theatre, a surgeon will have many other commitments. Those consultants with an interest in surgical research can choose to work in academic units. Consultants can also opt to have contracts with NHS trusts so that they can continue to work both in clinical practice and research. Those with academic intentions can be appointed as lecturers, senior lecturers or readers, perhaps leading subsequently to a chair (position of professor) in surgery. Other consultants spend some of their time in private practice and surgery can certainly be one of the more lucrative branches of medicine. As well as theatre time, consultants will need to run clinics and ward rounds and also spend an increasing amount of time undertaking managerial type roles. The duties of a surgeon are now formally outlined in a booklet published by the Royal College of Surgeons called *Good Surgical Practice.*

21.4 Training

The training programme in surgery is intensive. This may not suit those of us with other commitments and interests outside medicine. Flexible training can be arranged through the regional deaneries for those people who meet certain criteria. Other options include part-time training and job sharing. Obviously these programmes would involve more time spent at each level of the career pathway.

The surgical training pathway is currently undergoing significant change. Prior to 2005 the pathway from finishing medical school progressed through the pre-registration house officer (PRHO) year then the senior house officer (SHO) years during which the trainee would have to pass the MRCS examination to become a Member of the Royal College of Surgeons. The SHO years were known as basic surgical training years and would last a minimum of 2 years but sometimes several more. On completion of basic surgical training, a trainee applied for a post at the higher surgical training (HST) level in one of the surgical specialities listed in the box below. During this period the trainee would be a specialist registrar (SpR) and this period of training lasted for 5 or 6 years. After about 4 years of HST the trainee was eligible to take the intercollegiate speciality examination and this led to the award of the Fellowship of the Royal College of Surgeons (FRCS) diploma in the trainee's surgical speciality. At the end of this programme of training the trainee would gain CCST (Certificate of Completion of Specialist Training) and the qualified surgeon could then enter the General Medical Council's (GMC) Specialist Register and apply for a post as a consultant. There were several stages of competitive entry in this old programme and consequently trainees spent time enhancing their CVs (curricula vitae) in order to compete for their next promotion. Often trainees spent time in research or clinical posts that provided specialist experience. Many surgical trainees undertook a period of research for 1–3 years to obtain a higher degree (MSc, MD, MS, PhD) either before or during a higher specialist training (HST) programme.

From 2005 a new training programme has been initiated. All medical training is undergoing a radical transformation. These changes are currently evolving and up to date information is available on the Modernising Medical Careers (MMC) website (http://www.mmc.nhs.uk). Instead of PRHO posts, medical school graduates now proceed into a Foundation Year 1 (FY1) post (which will be similar to a PRHO post). They will then enter a second Foundation Year post

(FY2). These posts will provide broad training and trainees will have to demonstrate clinical competence and other work related skills which will be assessed in a number of different ways. The first new style trainees will finish their FY2 in August 2007. During the FY2 year trainees will have to make a decision about which area of medicine they want to pursue, not only broad areas such as hospital medicine or surgery, but specific specialities such as plastic surgery, urology or orthopaedics (see list in the box below). Trainees will have to choose 2 preferred areas of speciality and 2 regions of the country. If accepted onto a training programme the trainee will then spend the first 2 or 3 years in a variety of related specialities to their chosen field. During this period the trainee will be assessed on an annual basis. The trainee will then continue seamlessly into their HST in their chosen speciality for 3 or 4 years before being eligible to sit the speciality exam and complete their training. At this point trainees will be able to apply for a consultant post. The idea behind these changes is to streamline medical training so that once you are accepted to a training post, provided you successfully complete annual assessments, you will proceed to the consultant level without further competitive applications. This will shorten post-qualification training from 9 to 12 years to 7 or 8 years for surgical specialities.

Separate training programmes have been set up for those trainees that have an interest in an academic career. Those with an interest in research or teaching can apply following FY2 for an academic training post in their speciality of choice (medical, surgical or GP). This programme will contain similar clinical training but also dedicated protected time for research and teaching. Academic trainees will be expected to temporarily leave clinical training in order to do 3 years research for a PhD (or equivalent).

Surgical specialities

- *Breast*
- *Cardiothoracic:* heart and chest
- *General:* gastrointestinal system
- *Neurosurgery:* brain and spine
- *Oral and maxillofacial:* teeth and face
- *Orthopaedic:* bones and joints
- *Otolaryngology:* ear, nose and throat
- *Paediatrics:* children
- *Plastic surgery:* reconstructive, cosmetic
- *Urology:* kidney, bladder, prostate
- *Vascular:* blood vessels

21.5　The surgical exams and courses

The Membership of the Royal College of Surgeons (MRCS) examination is currently taken during the SHO years and will probably be taken in FY2 or the first years of subsequent training in the new system. Surgical trainees will also continue to be required to have successfully completed an approved basic surgical skills course (BSS). The MRCS is currently split into three parts. Parts 1 and 2 are multiple choice question (MCQ) papers. Part 3 comprises a viva voce (interview style exam) and clinical exam (examining patients and clinical information) this format will continue until at least 2010. Two other courses – the ATLS (Advanced Trauma and Life Support) and CCrISP (Care of the Critically Ill Surgical Patient) – are also recommended as part of training.

21.6　The job

One of the main preconceptions about surgery is that surgeons spend all their time operating. Generally speaking, this only occupies around a quarter of the working week. A surgeon will have patients on the ward, either waiting for their operation (preop), or having had the procedure carried out (postop). The surgeon will see these patients on a daily ward round. Another activity is seeing patients in the outpatients' clinic, where people who have surgical conditions are seen after being referred by their GP. We have outlined a typical day of a consultant surgeon below:

A day in the life of a consultant surgeon

The day usually starts at 8 am with a ward round. All the patients in hospital are under the care of a consultant, and surgery is not an exception. He or she will see the patients under his or her care and also those that have been admitted as emergencies. Management plans need to be decided for all the patients, which can then be carried out following the ward round. Some of the patients might be very unwell or require complex investigations. Other patients will have arrived that morning for routine or planned surgical procedures. Each of these patients will be seen before the operation. Some of the patients will be recovering after their operation, some staying for up to 2 weeks and some will be well enough to be discharged home.

On this day, after the ward round, the surgeon will go to the operating theatre for their list, which is likely to last around 3 hours. There will be patients having different types of operations, some short cases and some long and difficult procedures. The consultant will be assisted by other trainee surgeons on the team and one of the responsibilities is the training of these junior doctors.

After the operating list, during lunchtime, there is usually a meeting to attend. This could be a radiology meeting, where the X-rays of patients are reviewed, or possibly an audit meeting or teaching session.

This typical day involves an outpatient clinic in the afternoon. The clinic involves seeing patients, asking about their symptoms and examining them, and possibly making a diagnosis. The patient might then require surgery and be put on the waiting list, or might be treated with medications. You might have to tell a patient good or bad news depending on their condition and prognosis (outlook).

Every fifth night, you will need to be on call, where patients who are unwell are admitted to hospital, either referred from GPs or from the casualty department. The patients may be very sick and could require an urgent operation. This can be very hectic if lots of patients turn up at once. You will also have other responsibilities:

- teaching medical students and the other doctors on the firm;
- research – investigating new or existing modes and outcomes of surgery;
- audit – ensuring that the work being carried out in the hospital is being done to an acceptable standard;
- paperwork – such as writing notes, reports or letters to GPs and other doctors.

21.7 The options

Several decades ago, a surgeon was able to perform many different operations. It was not unusual for a surgeon to operate on breast, bowel, vascular and urological problems. In the modern era surgeons tend to be less general and focus on a particular area (a so-called speciality). Even the gastrointestinal tract has been split into smaller areas and it is common for a surgeon to become a specialist in either the upper or lower gastrointestinal operations.

21.8 Women in surgery

Women now make up 5% of consultant surgeons, 16% of surgery registrars and 24% of SHOs, and these numbers are growing. There is also a group called Women in Surgical Training (WIST), set up in September 1991 by The Royal College of Surgeons, whose aim is to promote surgery as a career for women. Their aim is to quadruple the number of female consultant surgeons by the year 2009.

21.9 Training abroad

Under the MRCS regulations only those posts approved by the Surgical Royal Colleges of England, Edinburgh, Glasgow and Ireland are recognised as entry requirements for the examination along with other posts stated in the regulations.

21.10 Flexible training

This is possible in surgery and is becoming more common, although less so than in other specialities within medicine. The training period must be approved by the specific royal college before commencement. You can get advice on flexible training from the College's flexible training advisor who can be contacted via the training board by letter, by email at: careers@rcseng.ac.uk or by telephone on: +44 (0) 20 74053474.

21.11 Further information

An excellent source of information is the surgical careers day held several times a year at the Royal College of Surgeons in London. There are guest speakers from every step of the surgical career pathway. Each speaker is then subjected to a question and answer session. The day concludes with a tour of the college and a surgical skills session. Each student also receives an information pack about CV skills and the career pathway.

21.12 The surgical specialities

Cardiothoracics

As the name suggests this field deals with the heart and chest and includes the famous coronary artery bypass grafting (to bypass blocked arteries that supply the heart), replacing heart valves, heart transplants, repairing inherited heart defects in children, and some operations for victims of chest trauma. The cardiothoracic surgeons also operate on the lungs. This is very demanding work. Most of the operations by their nature are carried out on people that are not very fit and this brings associated risks. Cardiothoracic surgeons work closely with the cardiologists (medical heart specialists) and respiratory physicians (lung specialists) who will refer patients for surgery and perform preoperative assessments and investigations. This is a challenging field of surgery which requires significant commitment.

ENT surgery/otolaryngology

ENT is the popular way of saying *otorhinolaryngology* – or head and neck surgery. Although you are working on just one small part of the body, there is a huge amount of skill required. The job involves repairing disorders of hearing, smell, taste, and speech and language. Although you will be performing a wide range of operations, there are also a lot of patients to be seen in the outpatient clinic. One of the joys of ENT is a chance to play with some of the weird and wonderful technology, such as microscopes and endoscope cameras to look into the body. A good ENT surgeon will be able to listen to patients' problems, have good management skills, good manual and technical skills and be able to work as part of a multidisciplinary team.

General surgery

A decade ago, a general surgeon would operate on the major blood vessels, the breast, and the bowels – quite a job. Now the speciality is subspecialising, but all surgeons still initially train in all those areas. Consultant general surgeons are usually practitioners in one of these subspeciality areas and also take responsibility for acute general surgical take. The practical elements and enjoyment of the practical tasks are probably the main attractions to any surgical speciality. The challenge is to perform the repeated practical task to an even higher degree of excellence. Nonetheless, skilful decision making about patient management and meticulous postoperative care also provide challenges and their own rewards. A good general surgeon will be able to undertake responsibilities, have good manual dexterity, good organisational ability and be physically fit!

Although the training to become a general surgeon is the same at the registrar level, most consultant surgeons then specialise in one area of:

- gastrointestinal (bowel) surgery
- breast surgery
- vascular surgery.

Gastrointestinal surgeons operate on conditions such as cancer of the colon or stomach ulceration. Many patients are admitted to hospital on call with problems such as a perforated bowel. These patients can become extremely unwell in a short period of time and, although medical management can help, an operation is usually necessary.

Breast surgeons deal with both benign and cancerous diseases of the breast, seeing patients in clinic and, following a biopsy, perform a relevant operation.

Vascular surgeons deal with blood vessel diseases, such as blockages and burst vessels. Again, many patients attend the hospital extremely unwell and require intensive treatment both before and after surgery.

Maxillofacial surgery

This is almost a separate field. Most hospital maxillofacial surgeons have dual qualifications in dentistry and medicine. Most have done a dentistry degree first and then want to pursue a career in more complex surgery around the mouth and face. These surgeons now overlap with ENT and plastic surgery to some degree. They also see trauma to the facial bones and perform more complicated dental procedures. Most dentists get some experience in a maxillofacial unit as part of their training.

Neurosurgery

Neurosurgeons operate on the nervous system, which encompasses both the brain and the spinal cord. They diagnose and treat a variety of diseases that can affect it. Neurological problems are common and make up to a quarter of all emergency hospital admissions. Neurosurgeons do not just operate; they also look after the intensive care unit (ITU) management and rehabilitation of patients with disorders affecting the brain and skull, spine, and nervous system. The subspecialities include spinal surgery, treatment for epilepsy and the care of children. Following recent advances in technology, for example in computed tomography (CT) and magnetic resonance imaging (MRI) scans, many more neurological conditions are curable, for example head trauma and spinal injuries. The qualities required are: a caring attitude, ability to work in a team, honesty, reliability, understanding of one's limitations, good communication skills and organisational ability.

Orthopaedic and trauma surgery

Elective orthopaedic surgery takes place in most district general hospitals, making it one of the largest of the specialities within surgery. The speciality has certainly seen significant changes in the last 2 decades, with the advent of new instruments and techniques, for example minimally invasive surgery. There is now a spectrum of subspecialities available, ranging from joint replacements in hips and knees to microvascular surgery. The speciality is well balanced with routine operating cases complemented by a large amount of trauma cases, which can be very exciting and rewarding. Working closely with other therapists (for example, physiotherapy) and other specialities makes this a dynamic subject. The last few years have also seen major developments in the management of trauma patients with an increasing number of injuries being treated operatively, enabling more rapid patient rehabilitation. The qualities required are good manual dexterity, ability to learn biomechanical and biological concepts, dedication and enthusiasm, good spatial awareness to cope with procedures under X-ray control, and teamwork.

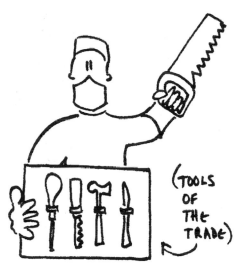

Career paths: orthopaedics

Paediatric surgery

This speciality involves a diverse workload that encroaches onto many other specialities, for example eyes, plastics and orthopaedic surgery. The main areas of surgery are trauma, intestinal and neonatal surgery. As a paediatric surgeon, you will work closely with GPs and other hospital doctors. There is limited opportunity for private practice. On-call commitments can vary but the emergency workload is interesting and never routine. It is a rewarding but busy career choice. Patience and good surgical techniques are required for this speciality, as are good communication and decision-making skills as you must support the parents as well as the child.

Plastic surgery

A broad-ranging speciality, which also assists many other specialities: cleft lip and palate surgery, breast reconstructive surgery, craniofacial surgery, limb reconstruction from either trauma or congenital abnormality, urogenital surgery in conjunction with the urologist (see below) and treating conditions of the skin. There is also cosmetic surgery, for example of the breast and face. Hand surgery can also form some of the workload, with a significant amount of congenital and traumatic problems. Plastic surgery is a truly dynamic speciality and encourages basic scientific and clinical research. The work is challenging, exciting and rewarding. A good plastic surgeon would have a high level of manual dexterity and technical skill, an enquiring mind and lateral

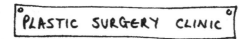

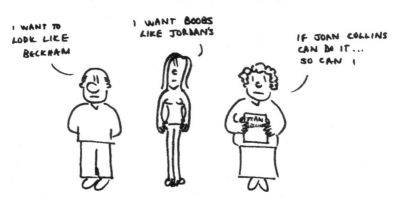

thinking ability and an understanding of the principles of audit and evidence-based medicine.

Urology

This is a very dynamic speciality involving the surgery of the kidney, bladder and genitourinary system. Many changes have occurred recently with the introduction of minimally invasive techniques. There is a good variety of emergency work and routine operating. Subspecialities include andrology (male hormone treatments), endo-urology (endoscopic treatments, that is, using probes and scopes), female urology, neuro-urology, oncological urology (cancer), paediatric urology and reconstructive urology. You will see patients with a wide breadth of pathology, including urinary tract stone disease, infections and malignancy. Three of the most predominant male cancers are urological: prostate, bladder and kidney cancers. In the younger male age group, testicular cancer is number one of this group of cancers. There is an interesting range of surgical skills required, both endoscopic (using probes and scopes) and open, and urology has lots of new technology in its repertoire. If people are particularly interested, they can also extend their practice outside conventional boundaries, for example performing transrectal (via the patient's bottom) ultrasound scans and biopsies. Because most departments are relatively small in respect of consultant numbers, there may be fairly frequent on-call sessions, but urology on call is not arduous and there is an increasing trend to cross-cover with neighbouring hospitals to reduce the on-call frequency. The qualities required are good patient and colleague communication, ability to work in a team, and good manual dexterity demonstrated by both open and endoscopic operative skills.

PERSONAL VIEW   *Sir Peter Morris*

Although I only decided to do medicine 6 months or so before I was due to go to university, I was quite sure, having made the decision to enter medicine rather than engineering, that I wanted to be a surgeon. To some extent this decision was influenced by reading a biography of Henry Cushing, the famous neuro-surgeon in Boston in the 1930s, and also to some extent by the fact that, as a good ball player, I liked doing things with my hands.

The 6 years at medical school at the University of Melbourne were the best years of my life. I was a reasonable student but had lots of interests outside med-icine. Nevertheless my ambition to be a surgeon never changed. After gradua-tion and completing my house jobs, I spent a further 3 years as a surgical resident at St Vincent's Hospital, Melbourne. It was during those several years that I had a lucky break. Dr Claude Welsh, a famous surgeon from the Massachusetts General Hospital (MGH) in Boston, came to St Vincent's as a vis-iting professor. In those days a visiting professor came for several months and operated most days on complex cases saved up for the great man by the sur-gical staff of the hospital. I was fortunate enough to be selected as his surgical registrar during his time in Melbourne, which meant that I was with him all day, every day, seeing patients, doing ward rounds and operating with him. He was an inspiration as a surgeon, never raised his voice, said please and thank you to everyone, even in the operating room, and yet achieved outstanding results in the complex surgical cases he had been asked to tackle. He was my ideal surgeon and the experience reinforced not only my resolve to be a sur-geon but also my concept of the ideal behaviour of a practising surgeon. After he left we kept in touch and several years later I was to go to the USA and the MGH at his request. My surgical training started in Australia, after which I went to the UK for just over 2 years before going to Boston, first as a senior resident in surgery and then as a junior staff man and research fellow at Harvard Medical School. As an aside, I did spend 6 months in general practice before leaving for the UK, in order to save some money for the trip, and I thoroughly enjoyed this experience.

I had an excellent training in the UK, both in London and especially in Southampton where I received an enormous amount of supervised operative experience under the tutelage of Mr Tom Rowntree. Moving to the USA was another major influence on my career, for not only did I learn within the huge department of surgery at the MGH that there were many ways of tackling a given operation, but also I was exposed to research for the first time. Initially I worked on the immunology of inflammation and infection but later switched

(Continued)

(Continued.)
to the immunology of transplantation, with a particular interest in tissue matching, a science in its infancy at that time. This experience made me sure that I wished to pursue a career in academic surgery, not only performing surgery but also doing research in areas of relevance to my clinical practice. Another lucky break followed when, just before I was due to return to Australia, I was asked by David Hume, the famous pioneer transplant surgeon, to join his department at Richmond, Virginia. Here he had established the largest transplant unit in the world at that time, and he wanted me to set up a tissue typing laboratory for the unit. This I did over a 7-month period as that was all the time I could give him before returning to Australia. This was another extraordinary experience in that I achieved what I had been asked to do but also was able to make some major contributions to the field of tissue matching using samples that Hume had preserved from the time of his first transplant.

On return to the University of Melbourne, I was a lecturer in the Department of Surgery with wide ranging clinical responsibilities in general surgery and transplantation. One must realise that in those days we were trained as true general surgeons. I also started the transplantation research laboratories and set up another tissue typing laboratory – the first in Australia. After a very successful and enjoyable 7 years in Melbourne, by which time I had gone from lecturer to senior lecturer and finally reader in surgery, I was invited to Oxford University as the Nuffield Professor of Surgery and Chairmanship of the department at the ripe old age of 39.

It was a great move in many ways as I was able to set up a transplant and vascular unit, the two specialities I eventually concentrated on. Research took off rapidly as six of my technicians came to Oxford with me, and so the laboratories were up and running quickly and the department never looked back.

So why be a surgeon? Certainly, if I had my time all over again, I have not the slightest doubt that I would do surgery once more. In surgical practice, in contrast to many other disciplines, you have the opportunity of curing a patient's problems by a properly selected and carefully done operation. There is nothing quite so rewarding!

Surgery has changed enormously over my career – many operations have disappeared completely as new medical treatments have appeared, for example, peptic ulcer surgery; many new operations have appeared, for example, laparoscopic cholecystectomy (removal of the gall bladder by keyhole surgery). I have no doubt that change will continue to occur, especially in the age of molecular biology, which will have an impact on surgical practice just as in medicine generally. But surgery will remain a marvellous discipline in which to specialise, particularly if you remember that a surgeon is a physician who operates!

Chapter 22 **Working abroad**

One worldwide inevitability is that people become unwell and require the services of medical professionals. This means it is frequently possible for doctors to travel and work in other parts of the world. The British medical degree seems to be fairly well respected around the world, with only the language barrier preventing work in many places.

In the past, taking time out from your training as a junior doctor was frowned upon and could have harmed your career progression. Currently, however, most consultants agree that working abroad can widen experience and it is considered more favourably. Increasing numbers of doctors are spending time during their junior years in foreign places. It is easy to understand the reasons: quite often it is possible to work in countries with better working conditions, enhanced pay and a better climate than in the UK.

After deciding to work abroad, you must then decide where, when and what to do. This involves researching the countries, hospitals and jobs, and talking to your senior colleagues as well as emailing and faxing potential hospitals. We list advantages and disadvantages of working abroad in the boxes below.

Advantages to working abroad

- Change of scene
- Cultural experience
- Opportunity to travel
- Meet new people
- Learn new skills
- Break from the career ladder
- Experience different healthcare system
- Experience different pathology

Disadvantages to working abroad

- Potential disruption to career path
- Leaving family and loved ones
- Problems applying and being interviewed for positions back home
- Organising the paperwork.

22.1 When to go – in the old days!

Traditionally the majority of medical graduates travelled abroad at some point during their first 2 years as a senior house officer. It was important to complete the pre-registration house officer (PRHO) year as most countries expected full registration with the General Medical Council (GMC). Most packed their bags immediately after finishing as a PRHO, and spent between 6 months and 2 years abroad (some stayed and never returned!). It was also possible to work abroad at other natural career breaks, i.e. between SHO (Senior House Officer) and SpR (Specialist Registrar) and SpR and consultant. It was also possible to spend part of your registrar training abroad and some doctors even took up locum consultant posts before settling into their speciality back home. There are a minority of practitioners that remain abroad, some meeting life-long partners and others finding the lure of the beach too great. The focus of this chapter is for those thinking of spending a short time in a different country. In summary, it was actually possible to work abroad during any part of your medical life but this did depend on your career choice and your examination timetable.

22.2 When to go – the future

With the introduction of modernising medical careers the timetable for working abroad may well change. The reality will probably mean that it will be harder to take time out of training, especially in the first few years of introduction of the new system. Due to the uncertain nature of the new application and job prospects, trainees are unlikely to risk their future career progression. This will no doubt change as the system beds in. What we do know is that it would be unwise for a trainee to leave for overseas before completing their foundation programme. There will be a natural break post foundation and this will probably be the most popular time for experience overseas to be gained. With the introduction of run-through training, the colleges should also allow doctors to train for at least part of their time in accredited jobs abroad. Although possibly a little more difficult than the current system, if you are keen to work abroad then the experience should be valuable so do go.

22.3 Where to go

There are two options: work in the western world, with similar technology and healthcare systems as the UK, or travel to a developing country. Colleagues choosing the latter have in general found themselves working more alone and at times with greater responsibility. The other big decision is whether to spend time in an English-speaking country or not. This will really depend on your language ability.

Europe

While it is possible to study in Europe, this will be extremely difficult without a firm grasp of the local language. The advantage of Europe is the proximity and the recognition of the British medical qualification. This means it is possible to work with confirmation of your competency provided by the GMC and without the need for a work permit. Language can be a problem; an A level in the subject is likely to be the minimal requirement necessary. Some doctors do attend language classes to assist them while abroad. While there are no formal language examinations, it is important to notify your future employers of your level of ability. Some hospitals do run exchange schemes and these are often advertised in the *British Medical Journal* (*BMJ*) careers section. The advantage of being from the UK is that, in most of the European countries where you might work, English is spoken fluently, and many of the medical journals are also published in English.

Australasia

The majority of UK graduates head off to seek warmer climates down under. With no language barrier, similar healthcare systems and plenty of adventure activities, it is easy to understand why. Certainly at SHO level, there are lots of opportunities, especially in emergency medicine and relief work (covering doctors on annual leave). At registrar level and above, it can be a little harder and it is often necessary to pass further local exams.

There are some differences that need to be noted. Firstly the grading of a doctor is slightly different. The hierarchy runs: consultant, registrar, RMO (Registered Medical Officer), and intern. The grade of registrar continues to be divided in Australia with junior registrars not requiring postgraduate examinations. This means that the registrar grade is similar to the SHO position in the UK and that some RMO posts can be more similar to PRHO. Doctors have gone to Australia and New Zealand under the impression that they will be commencing SHO equivalent posts, but have been disappointed by the lack of responsibility with the RMO jobs. Once postgraduate qualifications have been obtained, it is possible to become an advanced clinical trainee registrar, which is the equivalent of the SpR position in the UK.

(*Note*: Modernising medical careers is actually changing the training ladder so that the system is more like the current Australia model. When checking about the posts, discuss them in terms of years post graduation.)

The other main difference is the rota. Many hospitals are ahead of the UK when it comes to abolishing on call rotas and the majority of doctors will work full shifts. Instead of receiving a set wage, it is common practice to complete a time-sheet every 2 weeks. In this way a doctor gets paid for the actual hours worked, and so, if you are working nights or working a bank holiday, your pay reflects this.

USA

A much smaller number of graduates from the UK end up working in the USA compared to Europe and Australasia. Although there is no obvious language barrier, the healthcare systems differ and further examinations are required for the privilege. Most students who go to the USA have family connections and it is wise to make the decision to go early during your university years. The exams required are not straightforward and are divided into various sections. The qualification required is the USMLE (United States Medical Licensing Examination). Step 1 consists of basic medical sciences, with Step 2 involving clinical sciences (paediatrics, medicine, surgery, etc.). These can be taken during your university days and it is advisable to sit them during the relevant course when your knowledge will be greatest. The thought of covering the topics again later on is not appealing. Following the first two steps, it is now also necessary to complete a clinical exam, which actually takes place in the USA. Remember that funding for these exams will not be cheap.

Job allocation is done by a matching scheme, similar to that used by some of the universities in the UK. The jobs commence in July, which is not in line with British positions, and so could lead to some forced travel time or locum work. The other difficulty may be obtaining a visa and so advanced preparation is more essential than for moving to Australasia. As already mentioned, the healthcare systems are different, and so are working practices. The European Working Time Directive (as its name suggests) does not apply to the USA. The work may well be more intensive and working long hours is common. With private healthcare many patients have more extensive investigations to achieve a diagnosis. Less emphasis on bedside clinical skills and more reliance on technology can be disappointing for some clinicians as can the increased litigation that can ensue.

As the working practices differ across the Atlantic, it would be sensible to organise an elective placement in order to test the water. This will give you the opportunity to experience the American way before being committed to any contract or working future.

Preparation

Organising the trip can take several months and it is worth being well prepared. However, you might be able to sort out a job at fairly short notice and, from personal experience, this can be done in 2 months. Once a location has been decided, there are two choices – organise the job yourself or use an agency. Agencies can take a lot of the hassle out of finding a placement. Some of them have national interviews at certain times of the year in order to recruit. They offer incentives, such as free flights and insurance, but often the jobs are in more isolated locations, where recruitment has proved difficult from local graduates.

One of the easiest methods is to find the fax/email address of hospitals in the area where you would like to work (the Internet is a good starting point). Send a copy of your CV (curriculum vitae) with a covering letter to the medical staffing department and see what happens. It is always worthwhile making a follow up phone call to ensure they have received your CV and also to discuss opportunities in person. Medical staffing should then tell you the process of when the jobs become available and how to apply. Then you must finalise details of the actual job and salary. With the advent of the Internet some jobs are advertised on the web, either by the individual hospital or even by the regional health authority – in some instances it is possible to do a job search for the whole region for the particular speciality that appeals and then apply online.

Your future employer will require various documentations. Firstly check if the country you will be working in requires a visa. Again this can take some sorting, so it is worth considering early on. Most embassies issue visas by post but it can take 1–2 months. You also need to make sure your passport is valid for the full time you are abroad. Most developed countries will require evidence of your health status. This will, at the minimum, mean proof of your hepatitis status and other vaccines but you may also need a chest radiograph and HIV status. Don't forget that for some countries you may need further immunisations.

Travel insurance is necessary and each individual request will be different depending on length of stay, which country, possible procedures performed, accommodation type, etc. It is important to phone the company and get the product that suits best. A Certificate of Good Standing (states that no complaints have been made regarding your practice), available from the GMC, is requested by most employers. Copies of your actual GMC certificate, CV, references, and university degree may also be required (and original documentation can be asked for). Another factor to be considered is your NHS pension. Depending on your length of service, this may merely be frozen during your trip, but in some circumstances it may be cancelled. Contact the pension agency (through your employer) and explore the options. On arrival at your destination, you must register with the local medical board. Temporary registration is usually not a problem and your employer should have made them aware of your imminent arrival. Remember, all of the above will incur costs, so bear this in mind when budgeting and deciding on flight arrangements. Before leaving check with your indemnity insurance company that you will be covered abroad and make alternative arrangements if not.

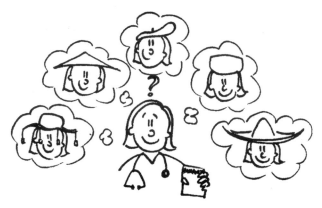

It is frequently possible for doctors to travel and work in other parts of the world

22.4 Voluntary work

If your debts are not too great and you feel like a different challenge, then consider voluntary work. Even though this is unpaid work, there is still competition for places with the larger organisations. One of the better known agencies is Medecins Sans Frontières. If you are accepted, work will normally be offered for approximately 12 months, and many of these groups send doctors to a great variety of destinations. Although there is no formal wage, set-up costs and living expenses will usually be covered. Other funding is often available for doctors wishing to spend time doing voluntary work. It is a case of trying as many different sources as possible. Write to local companies, charities, family, friends or even partake in a sponsored event.

Working abroad checklist

- Valid passport
- Relevant visa
- Immunisations
- Occupational Health Report
- Certificate of Good Standing
- Curriculum vitae

- Flights
- Travel insurance
- Indemnity cover
- Stethoscope
- *British National Formulary*

22.5 Other options

All work and no play may make for a dull life. Working abroad is a great opportunity to experience a different culture and many doctors spend some of their spare time travelling. Although previously frowned upon by potential employers, most now realise that time spent away can be useful and character building. It is not essential to work in a hospital or general practice while away. A minority fancy a more adventurous time and embark on journeys aboard cruise ships or even round the world yacht races. Most of us have heard of the flying doctors in Australia, but there are many less developed countries that also rely on these services. Information about these activities can be found on the Internet or in medical journals. To take part in sailing trips or mountain treks as the medical advisor will entail funding. This again has to be taken into consideration when taking account of your financial situation. Other companies may arrange working abroad seminars, so keep an eye out in the national journals.

22.6 Further information

It is often possible to organise your trip abroad single handedly. Most doctors travel with friends or partners but, if you are alone, do not be put off. Most of the hospitals in Australasia have large communities of British medical staff, many of whom have emigrated. The Internet is a vast source of knowledge for those arranging foreign travel and work. We have included some useful Internet addresses at the end of the book. Medical newspapers and journals also have jobs advertised. The other important point to remember is that, no matter where you have chosen to visit, other doctors will have been there before. Ask for their hints and tips and it may help you decide and also save some time.

Appendix

The following is a list of suggested websites where further information can be found. Where possible they are organised under the relevant chapter headings, although there will be overlap. We cannot guarantee the accuracy of the information on each site and do not endorse any of the products or services that may be offered. To gain the most from this list we suggest that you browse and select those areas that you find personally interesting – happy searching!

A challenging career
http://www.usitweb.shef.ac.uk/~mdb97djm/careers/apply.htm
http://www.baoms.org.uk/msg/HANDBK.HTM
http://www.dfes.gov.uk/studentsupport/
http://www.healthcentre.org.uk/hc/pages/student.htm
http://www.lmi.org.uk/6th_form_conference.htm
http://www.mcas.co.uk/
http://www.medlink-uk.com/
http://www.nhscareers.nhs.uk/nhs-knowledge_base/data/5343.html
http://www.premed.org.uk
http://www.roysocmed.ac.uk/academ/17-caree1.htm

The application procedure
http://www.asme.org.uk/compendium/courses.htm
http://www.entermedicine.co.uk
http://www.essaybank.co.uk/UCAS_Personal_Statements/Medicine/
http://www.gwydir.demon.co.uk/uklocalgov/
http://www.medschoolguide.co.uk/
http://www.support4learning.org.uk/careers/UK
http://www.ucas.com

The year out
http://www.bunac.org/
http://www.gap.org.uk/

http://www.gapwork.com/
http://www.gapyear.com/
http://www.gapyearjobs.co.uk/
http://www.missionafrica.org.uk/
http://www.payaway.co.uk/
http://www.projecttrust.org.uk/
http://www.springboard.co.uk/index.cfm
http://www.teaching-abroad.co.uk/
http://www.travellersworldwide.com/
http://www.work4travel.co.uk/
http://www.yearoutgroup.org/
http://www.yearoutgroup.org/organisations.htm

Choosing a medical school

Aberdeen: http://w3.abdn.ac.uk/medicine
Applying to Oxbridge:
http://www.cam.ac.uk/
http://www.ox.ac.uk/
Belfast: http://www.qub.ac.uk/cm
Birmingham: http://medweb.bham.ac.uk
Brighton and Sussex: http://www.bsms.ac.uk/home.html
Bristol: http://www.medici.bris.ac.uk
Cambridge: http://www.medschl.cam.ac.uk
Dundee: http://www.dundee.ac.uk/medicalschool/
Durham: see Newcastle
East Anglia: http://www.med.uea.ac.uk/
Edinburgh: http://www.med.ed.ac.uk/
Exeter and Plymouth: http://www.sasak.eurobell.co.uk/peninsula_
    medical_school.htm
Glasgow: http://www.gla.ac.uk/faculties/medicine/
Hull and York: http://www.hyms.ac.uk/
Keele: http://www.keele.ac.uk/depts/ms/
Leeds: http://www.leeds.ac.uk/medicine/
Leicester: http://www.le.ac.uk/medicine
Liverpool: http://www.liv.ac.uk/FacultyMedicine/
London:
Imperial College: http://www.fom.sk.med.ic.ac.uk/med/default.html
Kings College: http://www.kcl.ac.uk/depsta/medicine/
Queen Mary: http://www.mds.qmw.ac.uk/
St George's: http://www.sghms.ac.uk/
University College: http://www.ucl.ac.uk/medicine/

Manchester: http://www.medicine.man.ac.uk
Newcastle-upon-Tyne: http://www.ncl.ac.uk/undergraduate/subjects/med
Nottingham: http://www.nottingham.ac.uk/medical-school/
Oxford: http://www.medsci.ox.ac.uk/http://www.jr2.ox.ac.uk/
Sheffield: http://www.shef.ac.uk/~medsch/medsch.html
Southampton: http://www.som.soton.ac.uk/
St Andrews: http://biology.st-and.ac.uk/medsci/
Wales: http://www.uwcm.ac.uk/
Warwick: http://www.lwms.ac.uk/

The interview process
http://chemistry.about.com/library/weekly/aa013102a.htm
http://news.bbc.co.uk/1/hi/health/
http://www.health-news.co.uk/
http://www.newscientist.com/
http://www.qualitycvs.com/interviewtechnique.html
http://www.studentdoctor.net/index.asp

Over 21s
http://mwfonline.org.uk/medicalstudents.php
http://www.aber.ac.uk/mature/welfare.shtml
http://www.baoms.org.uk/msg/TRUSTMB.HTM
http://www.nhscareers.nhs.uk/nhs-knowledge_base/data/5343.html

Life at medical school
http://omni.ac.uk/browse/mesh/detail/C0038495L0038495.html
http://www.juiced.co.uk
http://www.nusonline.co.uk/
http://www.personal.u-net.com/~ic/fr_guide.html
http://www.studentbmj.com
http://www.studentcounselling.org/
http://www.studentdoctor.net/index.asp
http://www.studentfreestuff.com/
http://www.studentpages.com/
http://www.studentuk.com
http://www.ukcosa.org.uk
http://www.ukstudentguide.co.uk

The preclinical years
http://numedsun.ncl.ac.uk/~nds4/tutorials/
http://omni.ac.uk/browse/mesh/detail/C0038495L0038495.html

http://uia4.tripod.com/vol2/vol-No2_B3.html
http://www.drsref.com.au
http://www.fleshandbones.com/default.cfm
http://www.medal.org/
http://www.med.harvard.edu/AANLIB/home.html
http://www.medicalstudent.com/
http://www.medicalstudents.co.uk/links.htm
http://www.medshop.co.uk/
http://www.med.uiuc.edu/PathAtlasf/atlasindex.html
http://www.meduniv.lviv.ua/inform/studlinks.html
http://www.pastest.co.uk/pages/books/undergradbooksnormal.asp
http://www.stanford.edu/group/esource/MedicalStudent.html
http://www.studentdoc.com/
http://www.studentmedics.co.uk/
http://www.visembryo.com/

The clinical years
http://www.audrainmedicalcenter.com/ency/article/003137.htm
http://www.ecglibrary.com/ecghome.html
http://www.flash-med.com/Fact_Time.asp
http://www.medical-journals.com/
http://www.medical-sickness.co.uk
http://www.merck.com/
http://www.nottingham.ac.uk/pathology/medweb.html
http://www.radiology.co.uk/srs-x/index.htm
http://www.the-mdu.com/studentm/

The intercalated degree
http://usitweb.shef.ac.uk/~mdb97djm/careers/intercal.htm
http://www.medschool.com/futuretense_cs/MedSchool/faq/forums/
    intercalated.html
http://www.studentbmj.com/back_issues/1001/letters/393d.html
http://www.studentbmj.com/back_issues/1001/letters/393dres2.html
http://www.studentbmj.com/back_issues/1001/letters/393dres3.html
http://www.studentbmj.com/back_issues/1001/letters/393dres4.html

The elective
http://hpdrc.cs.fiu.edu/med.resource
http://www.emms.org/grants/elective.htm
http://www.healthserve.org/elecprep/contents.htm
http://www.medicine.man.ac.uk/som/HealthyElectives.ppt

http://www.medicsaway.co.uk/trips1.html
http://www.medicstravel.com/
http://www.rdinfo.org.uk
http://www.rsm.ac.uk/students/studprizedetail.htm
http://www.wellcome.ac.uk/en/1/biosfgcdpfunsumsep.html

Finances

http://www.dfes.gov.uk/studentsupport/uploads/finance2002.doc
http://www.missyourmum.com/money/instravel.shtml
http://www.moneynet.co.uk/student_index.shtml
http://www.slc.co.uk
http://www.studentfinancedirect.co.uk
http://studyfirst.direct.gov.uk/
http://www.studentmoney.org.uk/
http://www.direct.gov.uk/EducationAndLearning/
    UniversityAndHigherEducation/fs/en

Life as a junior doctor

http://money.guardian.co.uk/work/wageslaves/story/0,11996,714966,00.html
http://www.bma.org.uk
http://www.bma.org.uk/ap.nsf/Content/_Hub+jdc
http://www.doh.gov.uk/
http://www.doh.gov.uk/juniordoctors/
http://www.helpdoctor.co.uk/
http://www.medicalprotection.org/medical/united_kingdom/default.aspx
http://www.mwfonline.org.uk/
http://www.thedoctorscoach.co.uk
http://www.traineedocs.org.uk/

Career paths

Academic Medicine: http://www.chms.ac.uk/chms_pubs.html
Association for Palliative Medicine: http://www.palliative-medicine.org
Association of Anaesthetists: http://www.aagbi.org
Association of British Neurologists: http://www.theabn.org/
Association of Surgeons of GB and Ireland: http://www.asgbi.org.uk
British Association for A&E Medicine: http://www.baem.org.uk
British Association of Dermatologists: http://www.bad.org.uk
British Association of Occupational Therapists: http://www.cot.co.uk
British Atherosclerosis Society: http://www.britathsoc.ac.uk
British Cardiac Society: http://www.bcs.com
British Dietetic Association: http://www.bda.uk.com

British Medical Association: http://www.bma.org.uk
British Nuclear Medicine Society: http://www.bnms.org.uk
British Oncological Association: http://www.boaonline.org.uk
British Orthopaedic Association: http://www.boa.ac.uk
British Pharmacological Society: http://www.bps.ac.uk
British Renal Society: http://www.britishrenal.org/
British Society for Audiology: http://www.b-s-a.demon.co.uk/index.html
British Society for Endocrinology: http://www.endocrinology.org/
    default.htm
British Society for Geriatrics: http://www.bgs.org.uk/
British Society for Haematology: http://www.blacksci.co.uk/uk/society/bsh
British Society for Immunology: http://immunology.org/
British Society for Neurophysiology: http://www.bscn.org.uk/links.html
British Society for Rheumatology: http://www.rheumatology.org.uk/
British Society of Gastroenterology: http://www.bsg.org.uk
British Society of Rehabilitation Medicine: http://www.bsrm.co.uk/
British Thoracic Society: http://www.brit-thoracic.org.uk
    Diabetes UK: http://www.diabetes.org
Modernising Medical Careers: www.mmc.nhs.uk
RCP Faculty of Pharmaceutical Medicine: http://www.f-pharm-med.org.uk
Royal College of Anaesthetists: http://www.rcoa.ac.uk
Royal College of General Practitioners: http://www.rcgp.org.uk
Royal College of Obstetricians and Gynaecologists: http://www.rcog.org.uk
Royal College of Ophthalmologists: http://www.rcophth.ac.uk
Royal College of Paediatrics and Child Health: http://www.rcpch.ac.uk
Royal College of Pathologists: http://www.rcpath.org/contents.html
Royal College of Physicians: http://www.rcplondon.ac.uk
Royal College of Physicians of Edinburgh: http://www.rcpe.ac.uk
Royal College of Physicians & Surgeons of Glasgow: http://www. rcpsglasg.
    ac.uk/index.html
Royal College of Psychiatry: http://www.rcpsych.ac.uk
Royal College of Radiologists: http://www.rcrad.org.uk/
Royal College of Surgeons of Edinburgh: http://www.rcsed.ac.uk
Royal College of Surgeons of England: http://www.rcseng.ac.uk
Royal Society of Medicine: http://www.rsm.ac.uk
The Society of Occupational Medicine: http://www.som.org.uk/

Training as a general practitioner
Books for MRCGP: http://www.donfer.co.uk
Discussion Forum: http://www.nanp.org.uk
GP recruitment: http://www.gprecruitment.org.uk/

Postgraduate training: http://www.jcptgp.org.uk/
Postgraduate training: http://www.postgradgpliv.com/
Preparation course: http://www.mrcgpexam.co.uk
Summative assessment: http://www.nosa.org.uk/

Training in the medical field

1200 MCQs for MRCP Part I: http://www.mrcppart1.co.uk/mcqs.php3
Case Database: http://medweb.bham.ac.uk/http/caa/cases/
Clinical signs: http://www.users.dircon.co.uk/~rosebud/mrcp/_frame.html
Exam discussion groups: http://www.mrcppart1.co.uk/mcqs.php3
MRCP site: http://www.mrcpuk.org/
On examination - MRCP Part I: http://www.onexamination.com
Revision courses: http://www.mrcppart1.co.uk/course.php3
Royal College of Physicians: http://www.rcplondon.ac.uk/index.asp
Tips: http://www.dundee.ac.uk/medicine/MRCP/mrcpuk1tips.htm
Useful Stuff: http://www.chills.co.uk/
Viva booklets online: http://praxis.md/

Training in the surgical field

Exam Info: http://www.rcseng.ac.uk/surgical/examinations/
News – to help with viva: http://www.surgical-tutor.org.uk/journals.htm
Online Tutorials: http://www.surgical-tutor.org.uk/tutorial.htm
Pathology Database: http://www.surgical-tutor.org.uk/pathhome.htm
Regulations for MRCS at RCPS Glasgow: http://www.rcpsglasg.ac.uk/
    regulations.htm
Revision notes: http://www.surgical-tutor.org.uk/revision.htm
Surgeons-Tutor: http://www.surgical-tutor.org.uk/mcqhome.htm
X ray Database: http://www.surgical-tutor.org.uk/xrayhome.htm

Working abroad

http://international.monster.com/workabroad/articles/health/
http://www.babelfish.altavista.com:
http://www.doctorsoftheworld.org/
http://www.fco.gov.uk/travel
http://www.holtmedical.com/workingabroad.htm
http://www.masta.org/
http://www.mediwork.info/

Medical resources

Agency for Healthcare Policy: http://www.ahcpr.gov/
Audit Commission: http://www.audit-commission.gov.uk

Best Medical Resources on the Web: http://www.priory.co.uk/othermed.htm

British Library Information Service: http://www.icarus.bl.uk/sris/irs.html

Centre for Evidence-based medicine: http://cebm.jr2.ox.ac.uk/

Clinical Governance: http://www.le.ac.uk/cgrdu

Department of Health: http://www.doh.gov.uk

Doctor Online: http://www.doctoronline.nhs.uk

Doctors.net: http://www.doctors.net.uk/

Doctorsworld.com: http://www.doctorsworld.com/

Draft template of audit risk management report: http://www.doh.gov.uk/ntro/risktemp.html

Equip Magazine: http://www.equip.ac.uk/index.html

General Medical Council: http://www.gmc-uk.org/

Health and Safety Executive (HSE): http://www.hse.gov.uk/hsehome.htm

Health Education Authority: http://www.hea.org.uk

HealthEconomics.Com: http://www.exit109.com/~zaweb/pjp

Index of registered medical research charities: http://bubl.ac.uk/uk/charities/med.htm

InteliHealth: http://www.intelihealth.com/IH

Internet GratefulMed: http://igm.nlm.nih.gov/

Links to government websites: http://www.tagish.co.uk/tagish/links/

Medical Audit.co.uk: http://www.medicalaudit.co.uk

Medical Devices Agency: http://www.medical-devices.gov.uk

Medical Info Search: http://www.pavilion.co.uk/mednet/find_med.html

Medical Resource Reviews Database: http://www.hpdrc.cs.fiu.edu/med.resource

Medical Matrix: http://www.medmatrix.org/reg/login.asp

Medical Resource Database: http://www.hpdrc.fiu.edu/med.resource/

Medical School Info: http://www.chms.ac.uk/

Medical Search Engine: http://www.achoo.com/main.asp

Medical Search Tools: http://wwnurse.com/medsearch.shtml

Medical Women's Federation: http://www.mwfonline.org.uk

MedWebPlus: http://www.medwebplus.com

National Audit Office: http://www.nao.gov.uk/

National Network of Libraries of Medicine: http://nnlm.gov

NHS Centre for Evidence-Based Medicine: http://www.priory.co.uk/othermed.htm

NHS Confederation: http://www.nhsconfed.co.uk/

NHS Direct Online: http://www.med.monash.edu.au/shcnlib/dehsj

NHS Workforce Development Confederations: http://www.wdc.nhs.uk

NICE. http://www.nice.nhs.uk

NPC – Audit handbook: http://www.npc.co.uk

PRODIGY: http://www.prodigy.nhs.uk/
PubMed (Medline): http://www.ncbi.nlm.nih.gov/PubMed/
Royal Medical Benevolent Fund: http://www.rmbf.co.uk/
SciTech Resources: http://www.scitechresources.gov
SHOW (Scottish Health on the Web): http://www.exit109.com/~zaweb/pjp
Silver Platter Information: http://www.intelihealth.com/IH

Health informatics
Health informatics journal: http://www.shef-ac-press.co.uk/hij.htm
Health information on the Internet: http://www.hioti.org
Informatics Review: http://www.informatics-review.com

Medical statistics
Hospital inpatient data: http://www.doh.gov.uk/hes
Hyperstat Online: http://davidmlane.com/hyperstat/
    index.html
Medical statistics on the web: http://www.gla.ac.uk/Library/Depts/
    MOPS/Stats/medstats.html
Statistical calculators: http://members.aol.com/johnp71/javastat.html
Statistics at Square One: http://www.bmj.com/collections/
    statsbk/index.shtml
Stats Direct: http://www.camcode.com

CHMS documents
The Council of Heads of Medical Schools and Deans of UK Faculties of
Medicine was originally established in Jan 1992. They have published a variety
of useful documents:

A survey of clinical academic staffing levels in UK
Equal opportunities for medical students: http://www.chms.ac.uk/
    chms_pubs.html
Medical and dental schools: http://www.chms.ac.uk/chms.pdf
Medical education and research: http://www.chms.ac.uk/chms_pubs.html
Nursing education: http://www.chms.ac.uk/chms_pubs.html
Research assessment: http://www.chms.ac.uk/chms_pubs.html
Responses to government papers: http://www.chms.ac.uk/chms_pubs.html
Student health and conduct: http://www.chms.ac.uk/chms_pubs.html

Index

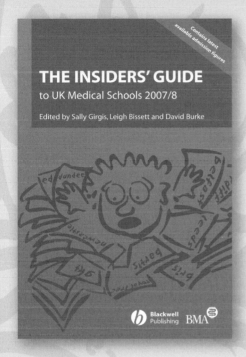
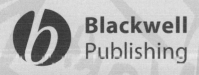
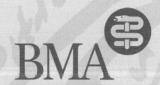